Conventional Cancer 'Cures' – What's the Alternative?

A Comprehensive Guide to
Cancer Therapies
from around the World

Chris Woollams

Copyright © 2004 Chris Woollams and Health Issues Ltd

Chris Woollams asserts the moral right to be identified as the editor and author of this complete work.

A catalogue record for this book is available from the British Library.

All rights reserved. No part of this book may be reproduced or transmitted in any form or by any means, electronic or mechanical, including photocopying, recording, or by any information storage retrieval system, without permission in writing from the publisher and the author.

First published in January 2005 by:
Health Issues Ltd
The Elms, Radclive Road, Gawcott, Buckingham, MK18 4JB
Tel: 01280 815166
Fax: 01280 824655
E-mail: enquiries@iconmag.co.uk

Cover design by Jeremy Baker

ISBN 0-9542968-7-7

Printed in Great Britain by Bath Press Ltd, Lower Bristol Road, Bath BA2 3BL

Important notice

This book represents a review and an interpretation of a vast number of various sources available to anyone on the subject of cancer. Articles have been prepared by the author himself and a number of others from professors and medical experts to professional journalists and nutritionists. The book is merely designed to save the reader time in their quest for information.

Whilst the author has made every effort to ensure that the facts, information and conclusions are accurate and as up to date as possible at the time of publication, the author and publishers assume no responsibility.

The author is neither a fully qualified Health Practitioner nor a Doctor of Medicine and so is not qualified to give any advice on any medical matters and nor will he do so. Cancer (and its related illnesses) is a very serious and individual disease, and readers must consult with experts and specialists in the appropriate medical field before taking, or refraining from taking, any action.

Such specialist advice should always be sought for accurate diagnosis and before any course of treatment.

The author and the publisher cannot be held responsible for any action, or lack of action, that is taken by any reader as a result of information contained in the text of this book. Such action or lack of action is taken or not taken entirely at the reader's own risk.

In loving memory of Catherine

In the middle of the journey of our life I came to myself within a dark wood where the straight way was lost.

Dante Alighieri (1265–1321),
The Divine Comedy

Contents

	Introduction	xi
1	**Cancer cells are different** *Chris Woollams*	1
2	**Could you eat yourself well?** *Chris Woollams*	5
3	**California dreamin'** *An interview with Charlotte Gerson by Chris Woollams*	13
4	**Eat to beat cancer?** John Boik – a total attack on cancer by natural compounds *Chris Woollams*	21
5	**Natural Progesterone** *Chris Woollams*	25
6	**Attack of the enzymes - the pancreas strikes back** (Beard, Kelley and Gonzalez therapies) *Chris Woollams*	33
7	**Can one diet fit all?** *Chris Woollams*	41
8	**Blood typing** *Ginny Fraser*	45
9	**Metabolic typing** *Ginny Fraser*	53
10	**"There are no rules" – keeping an open mind** *An interview with Dr Etienne Callebout by Ginny Fraser*	61
11	**B-17: 'Nature's chemotherapy'** *Chris Woollams*	69

12	**Mexican wave** *An interview with Dr Francisco Contreras* Chris Woollams		75
13	**Metabolic therapy and the causes of cancers** Dr Paul Layman		85
14	**C for yourself** (an article on the benefits of vitamin C) Chris Woollams		95
15	**Are there safer ways of killing cancer cells than chemotherapy?** (Vitamin C megadoses) Dr Julian Kenyon		105
16	**A review of key vitamins and minerals. But do they work on cancer?** Chris Woollams		109
	(a)	Vitamin A	109
	(b)	Beta-carotene	115
	(c)	Vitamin B-12	119
	(d)	Vitamin D	123
	(e)	Vitamin E	128
	(f)	Vitamin K	132
	(g)	Selenium	135
	(h)	Zinc	139
	(i)	Magnesium	142
17	**What else could help me?** Chris Woollams		145
	(a)	Glycoproteins and medicinal mushrooms	145
	(b)	MGN-3	149
	(c)	Aloe Vera	152
	(d)	Noni juice	155
	(e)	Chlorella	158
	(f)	Essiac	161
	(g)	Hoxsey – the quack that cured cancer?	165
	(h)	Hydrazine sulphate	170
	(i)	Coral calcium	174
	(j)	Mistletoe	175
	(k)	Carctol	177

18	**Can Candida cause cancer?** *Chris Woollams with Gerald Green*	181
19	**Things that go bump in the night** *Chris Woollams*	189
20	**Testing times** (a) **Vega testing** *Dr John Millward*	193 193
	(b) **The information highway of complementary medicine** *David Broom*	199
21	**Zap that cancer** *Ginny Fraser*	205
22	**A virus at the heart of every cancer?** *Chris Woollams on Dr Royal Rife*	211
23	**Using viruses to treat cancer** *Chris Woollams*	223
24	**Recharging your failing cells** The work of David Walker *Chris Woollams*	227
25	**Living in harmony** *Melanie Hart*	233
26	**What caused your cancer?** Dowsing for answers *Elizabeth Brown*	239
27	**Disrupting the power stations of brain tumours** *Professor Geoffrey Pilkington*	247
28	**A new approach to cancer treatment – can Phenergan treat cancer?** *Dr Robert Jones*	253

| 29 | **Photodynamic therapy**
Chris Woollams | 271 |

| 30 | **Dendritic cell therapy vaccines**
Dr Julian Kenyon | 281 |

| 31 | **Antineoplastons – a non-toxic treatment for cancer?**
The work of Dr Stanislaw Burzynski
Chris Woollams | 289 |

| 32 | **Hands on healing**
Madeleine Kingsley | 295 |

| 33 | **The power of prayer**
Ginny Fraser | 301 |

| 34 | **'John of God'**
Catherine Woollams | 307 |

Appendices:
1. **Parallel reading** — 315
2. **Contacts** — 317
3. **Contributors** — 323

Introduction

> "If the world should blow itself up, the last audible voice would be that of an expert saying, it can't be done."

I start my fifth book with the late Peter Ustinov's words and, in fact although they are the first words in the book, they are the last I wrote. Having read about so many devoted people who have dedicated their lives to helping people with their cancers, yet found their work an up-hill struggle, often ridiculed or completely dismissed, the quote seems most apposite.

Yet this book is my most important book. It is a level above all the others and aims quite simply to tell you, in some detail, about the best alternative and complementary therapies around the world. As such it is really Part II to my original 'best seller', *Everything you need to know to help you beat cancer*. If that original book was GCSE 'O' level then this is the university degree course!

This is a book that's not really a book. And I make no excuses. In fact, it is more like a patchwork quilt, largely comprised of a number of important articles that have run in **icon** (Integrated Cancer and Oncology News) magazine over the last 18 months and not always from my hand, with a good number of extra and important chapters added. You may find some chapters a little repetitive – overlapping – but I wanted each to give you the full unedited picture as originally written. As always, it is meant to be a really 'easy' read. However, judging by the telephone calls we receive daily in our offices, its importance to people touched by cancer cannot be stressed enough. This book should save everyone touched by cancer a lot of hard work.

As many people know my daughter had a grade 4 brain tumour.

Initially I was told – off the record – that she had 6 months to live. That was over three and a half years ago. The maximum anyone has lived in this condition is 18 months. We have tried to help her with all manner of complementary therapies and she has had the best treatment orthodox medicine can offer. Her surgeon has been excellent, absolutely first-class, but the chemotherapy has completely failed, not that I expected anything else. Only recently the *Lancet* ran an article clearly stating that drugs do not work for brain tumours (Feb. 2004). The drugs, as is often the case, did however make her very ill indeed.

Doctors told her there was not a lot more they could do.

But I had been researching this subject for almost every hour of every day for three years and I knew there are treatments – not 'quack' hocus-pocus remedies – but **real** treatments that have cured others when the chips were down. And for Catherine we reviewed and used some of the best of them. At one point her oncologist said to her face that "he hadn't expected her to still be around"! For a while some of these treatments undoubtedly helped.

When we launched the first book *'Everything you need to know to help you beat cancer',* we did it simply because we believed other people touched by cancer should have access to all the basic information I had discovered in my early attempts to help Catherine, so they might also improve their chances of beating the disease. Put simply *Everything you need to know to help you beat cancer* was meant to be the basic bible – the fount of knowledge – providing easy to read information to save you at least six months hard work. We continued this theme when we launched **icon** (Integrated Cancer and Oncology News) magazine; now freely available in more than one hundred top hospitals and oncology units every two months. We research treatments properly and tell the **whole** truth about **all** these treatments so people touched by cancer can make **informed decisions**. Our charity **CANCERactive** supports this with a mission to provide **information** for both prevention and cure.

Introduction

And so we come to this book, our patchwork quilt. Again, we are merely passing on information to people. Information you have a right to know. Information that will save you a year or two of your own in research. A year or two you might not have without the information.

Do the therapies in this book work? Do radiotherapy and chemotherapy actually cure cancer? Now, there's a debate that would take a whole book in itself.

Conventional cancer 'cures' from our hospitals tend to be limited to just surgery, radiotherapy and chemotherapy: What I call the unholy trinity. Certain open-minded specialists do broaden their options. The Royal Marsden is handing out vitamin D and doing work on Red Clover with breast cancer patients for example. But, by and large, medical authorities seem to be intent on restricting options rather than expanding them. Surely this runs counter to almost any other scientific area you care to look into? And, dare I add, to the latest UK Government initiative for patients, namely 'choice'.

Yet chemotherapy historically has been all but useless in cases of pancreatic cancer, brain tumours, multiple myeloma and a number of other cancers. One specialist told me that radiotherapy on its own only had a 15 per cent success rate. Is it any wonder that total 5-year survival rates have only improved by 12 per cent over the last 30 years according to a recent report by the National Audit Office (UK-2004, Feb)?

Then there are the side effects. The weakening of the immune system during surgery, radiotherapy and chemotherapy just when you need it to be strong. The loss of hair, or nails, the nausea, tiredness and depression.

Some people faced with cancer simply don't want to go through all this. Some people feel there must be a better way.

Even surgery, experienced by 60 per cent of patients, has its doubters; and not just amongst patients. Some doctors feel it may even spread the cancer it seeks to eradicate! There have even been learned articles in The Lancet highlighting this concern.

I have recently seen pictures of algae and chlorophyll derivatives that target cancer and pre-cancer cells in the body illuminated by special 'light' machines. Women with 'a tumour' in their breasts, in fact had ten or so 'hot spots' **all over their body**. How would surgery combat this? Worse, women who had had chemotherapy already had many, many more hot spots around their bodies probably indicating an extra weakness to resist the cancer by cells throughout the body compromised by the toxic effect of chemotherapy. And on the debate over surgery, the pictures show bands of cancerous and pre-cancerous cells down the incision lines on ovarian cancers. All oncologists should see these pictures.

Add to this the statement by the prestigious MD Anderson Cancer Center that "all the exciting developments in cancer treatment are coming in areas outside chemotherapy" and I worry that the medical profession in the UK, almost lemming-like, might be galloping towards a cliff. Unfortunately they are taking us, the general public, with them.

Please be absolutely clear. I, personally, never offer advice – I just pass on information. Equally, we make no claims about curing cancer. We just genuinely believe that there are a number of things every cancer patient can do to increase their odds of a longer, more personally fulfillng survival.

The saddest fact is that I genuinely believe there are a number of simple things you can do to improve your chances of beating cancer. Yet when these are mentioned, there are some people who immediately criticise and protest. If I said that my research had led to my 'discovery' of something that could reduce the number of cancer cases in Britain by up to 35,000 per year and the number of cancer deaths by up to 50,000 you might doubt me, but you'd certainly be interested. Unfortunately the medical profession don't share this view.

Introduction

The simple fact is that American Scientists took 38,000 people in a region with quite high rates of cancer in China, and conducted a 5-year test prior to 1993. The people were given various antioxidants daily but at levels of only twice the RDA (Recommended Daily Allowance), which is still a small dose. Indeed for vitamin C at this small level there was no benefit. But in one sub-test, the group taking twice the RDA of beta-carotene, vitamin E and selenium showed a 13 per cent decrease in the number of cancer cases and 21 per cent fewer deaths in just those five years.

Critics might say, "it was China", or "a one off experiment" but a similar study, the Su.Vi.Max study, finished in France in the autumn of 2003. There, 17,000 people took a five-antioxidant supplement (selenium, zinc, vitamins E and C and beta-carotene) over seven years. The result? 31 per cent fewer men's cancers and 37 per cent fewer deaths. You'd expect the authorities to be jumping for joy.

But the French authorities were still saying that they best solution was to eat properly. Whilst we don't deny that is the best option, the fact is that people in general, proven by these 55,000 people in the two tests, don't. For them, the supplements saved lives. When will the governments and medical authorities wake up? Modern life is not about 'eating properly'. It's about jumping on planes, business meetings, food on the move, McDonalds, refined wheat, dairy, sugar, too much salt and so on. It's about mobile phones, toxic toiletries and radiation too. And if government and medical authorities are not prepared to attend to these core problems and issues, why are they so resolute in their attacks against research-proven simple anti-cancer measures, like antioxidant supplements?

Only recently the American Cancer Society has published a report looking at people who had taken 4 or more 'doses' of multivitamins per week in the 1970's. By the year 2000 this group had 30 per cent less colon cancer.

Did Western governments immediately send out a circular to health authorities on these 'amazing, breakthrough' vitamin and antioxidant findings? Did doctors and hospitals immediately notify the general population and their cancer patients with the wonderful news?

Why not? These figures are dramatic both for prevention and survival rates.

As I prepared this book it was hard, in fact, to keep an open mind. Stories on Burzynski, on Joseph Gold, Royal Rife and David Walker are genuinely alarming. These are professors and doctors who want to cure people; who have points of view and contributions to make. But instead of participating in open-minded debate, authorities in the USA just rush to shut them down. Business doesn't rush to shut down a Branson or a Bill Gates when they dare to say something different. Why is it thus with medicine?

Nor are we immune in the UK. Only recently in January 2004, some UK scientists conducted a simple research study of patients taking supplements. However, in the report they went on to criticise these 'Complementary Alternative Medicines' listing negative findings as old as 1979 or one-off studies whilst ignoring hundreds of more recent studies on their benefits. This report was actually published in the British Journal of Cancer for all scientists and doctors to see. So-called 'Complementary Experts' repeat the attacks on supplements. Statements like "Some Complementary Alternative Medicines can cause bleeding" were contained in the report. If a researcher working for my company in my advertising days had written this sort of unilateral statement, he or she would not have been employed very long! Imagine if we wrote in **icon**, 'some chemotherapy may cause bleeding or even death'! Would **icon** be even allowed in hospitals the following month?

Worse, it is quite clear to a number of scientists that understanding how vitamins (like K and D) help the anti-cancer process is very much in its infancy. Discoveries since the year 2000 for vitamin K with liver and leukaemia have added a whole new dimension to these almost unknown vitamins.

At least now in the USA the National Center for Complementary and Alternative Medicines has been formed and this has effectively silenced the more blatantly biased attacks, those who make wild and unsubstantiated comments against such alternative and complementary therapies. This has driven the critics underground. 'Quackwatch' for example, can only operate on the Web, and is largely discredited since its authors launched attacks on treatments like acupuncture. Are people really so worried that someone might discover a simple, cheap, non-toxic 'cure' for cancer?

Sadly, of course, they are. Dr Contreras tells the story of treating a US senator at his clinic in Mexico. On the last day the Senator asked him what he'd like to achieve in his life. "More effective results against child cancer; and, of course, I'd like to create the cure for cancer", was his reply. To this the Senator simply said, "If you went to the President of America tomorrow with the cure for cancer, you'd be dead within two days. Cancer is very big business, and without that business there would be widespread unemployment, stock market decline and huge reverberations throughout the Western world."

And so we come back to this little book, *Conventional Cancer 'Cures' – What's the Alternative?*

We do assume that you have probably read my first book, *Everything You Need to Know to Help You Beat Cancer*, and so understand the fundamentals of cancer, its causes and possible 'cures'. It was always intended as a 'kiddies guide', a 'bible' of the basics. This new book is intended as the follow-up. The patchwork quilt that can save you a year or two of research when time is not on your side. No promises, no guarantees. Just a collection of articles that show you there are alternatives and there are a number of great doctors and scientists making ground-breaking discoveries all the time. Be warned though. In the UK national press in May 2004 certain 'complementary experts' were stating that all such anti-cancer claims for complementary and alternative treatments were 'Bogus'. Decide for yourself.

And as we review more therapies over the coming year or so, I promise they will be included in any follow-up editions of this book, and put on our website (www.iconmag.co.uk).

Meanwhile my thanks, indeed indebtedness, to all those people who have contributed to **icon** and whose work appears in this book, including: Professor Geoff Pilkington, Dr John Millward, David Broom, Dr Julian Kenyon, Dr Robert Jones, Elizabeth Brown, Dr Paul Layman, Madeleine Kingsley, Ginny Fraser, Catherine Woollams, Melanie Hart and Maggie Goodman, plus the 'interviewed': Gerald Green, Charlotte Gerson, Dr Etienne Callebout, Dr Francisco Contreras, Dr David Walker and Dr William Porter. A share of the profits of this book will go to CANCERactive, our charity.

And finally, thanks to Lindsey Fealey, Janet Howatson and Karen Holden who had to put up with me as I completed it all.

Chris Woollams

1 Cancer cells are different

Chris Woollams

Let us be quite clear, right from the outset. **Cancer cells are different**.

Cancer cells resemble very primitive cells. During the first 56 days of a foetus in the womb the original fertilised cell divides extremely rapidly and all cells at the outset seem identical and undifferentiated. They are called stem cells. Stem cells seem to be switched on by the hormone, oestrogen, to form trophoblast cells. These are useful in, for example, the healing process, or after conception when the embryo needs to attach to the uterus wall and the placenta needs to develop. Then, as if a switch is turned on, these cells start to change multiplying at a slower, normal rate. Some become eye cells, or liver cells, or toe cells or lung cells. This is called differentiation. Unfortunately, sometimes the undifferentiated cells do not turn off after completing the job. Cancer cells are like the undifferentiated cells, dividing at a much faster rate than the normal differentiated cells surrounding them and never dying.

All cells contain power stations, called mitochondria. Normal cells take carbohydrate and burn it in the presence of oxygen in a long multi-step process to make your energy. The waste is excreted.

Cancer cells do not use oxygen. In fact its presence kills them. Otto Warburg won a Nobel Prize for this finding in 1931. Cancer cells also use glucose as their favourite food, and in a very short and less efficient process make their energy, excreting a waste product called lactic acid.

Lactic acid can only be detoxified by the liver. The end product of the detoxification is glucose, which in turn feeds the cancer providing a self-fuelling downward spiral. Cancer cells are very clever and thrive on the biological systems of the host, rather like a parasite. Some cancer treatments try to deliver oxygen into the cell to kill it. Some treatments limit glucose; others clean the liver or try to stop the recycling process.

The cancer energy production system features certain enzymes (the stimulators of chemical reactions) unique to a cancer cell and not normally found in a healthy cell. Some cancer treatments can target these unique enzymes.

Cancer cells produce much lower energy, than normal cells. This lower 'voltage' works like a battery running out of 'charge' and some of the protective mechanisms of the cell (the genes which repair any problems and keep it 'normal') are switched off. However, the genes that tell it to divide vigorously still work. Some treatments try to recharge the cells back to normal levels.

Cancer cells don't normally die. Some cancer treatments (for example the use of virology) try to induce death in them, while others try to turn them 'normal' so that they can die of old age.

The basic blueprint of the cell, the DNA, has been structurally altered so it is unlike the blueprint of the normal cells. Some cancer treatments target this change in the blueprint.

The body's immune system usually recognises 'foreign' cells like viruses, bacteria or emerging cancer cells and can neutralise them. Sometimes the immune system is too weak to neutralise the cancer cells. Some cancer treatments simply aim to boost the immune system.

Sometimes the cancer cells can hide from the immune system and it fails to recognise them as different. Some cancer treatments aim to re-stimulate this recognition process.

Sometimes toxins, or free radicals damage the cell. They punch holes in the outer membrane destroying the energy levels, or block receptor sites that transmit healthy messages. Or worse they block or attack the blueprint and its messages inside the cell causing a new rogue or abnormal cell to form, or rogue messages to be emitted. Some cancer treatments try to clean up this mess.

Sometimes the normal cell is damaged by simple everyday things. Too much salt (sodium) can enter the cell and particularly the power stations, displacing the normal mineral used, potassium. This causes the power stations to be less efficient, produce a more acidic environment and use less oxygen – setting up the situation that prevails in a cancer cell. Some cancer treatments try to clean up the diet to reinstate the correct mineral balance for a healthy cell.

Sometimes too much oestrogen is present in the body. This may turn on the production of 'trophoblast cells' or may depress oxygen in the power stations, both setting up the cancer situation. Some cancer treatments attempt to reduce the excesses of oestrogen in the body.

Cancer cells divide rapidly, making identical copies of the rogue original. This cluster grows and grows, occasionally firing some cells off into the blood or lymph systems. These travelling rogue cells may be mopped up by the immune system. Or they may collect in a lymph node or in another organ like the liver, lung or brain, where they form a secondary growth. This action is called metastasis. Some cancer treatments try to stop this 'spreading' activity.

The original cluster grows rapidly, but as it grows bigger it needs adequate nourishment to support the growth and division of new cancer cells. Such tumours need a blood supply. It provides nourishment whilst limiting the access of oxygen to the cells. Some cancer treatments attempt to disrupt this blood supply and thus the tumour.

Some tumours protect themselves by forming a protective protein coat around them. In this way, attacking agents from the immune system or chemotherapy drugs have difficulty reaching the rogue cancer cells. Some cancer treatments attempt to break down the protective coat.

Although a tumour may be localised, its causes and effects are seen throughout the body whether they are low oxygen, poor immune system, acid body, hormone imbalance or whatever. Some treatments try to clean up and rebalance the whole body. Some literally re-energise it.

Many cancer treatments, orthodox, complementary or alternative, are well researched. At **icon** we have no remit to support any particular form of treatment over any other. We just want to inform, to present all treatments that have merit and have research to prove it. You have a right to know about them all.

Sometimes however, scientific fact comes second to belief. In a major cancer hospital in the USA an analysis of the records of all cancer patients has shown that those with a God survive up to seven times longer than those without.

Much remains unknown about cancer cells!

2   Could you eat yourself well?

An overview by Chris Woollams

The World Health Organisation has stated that of the 6 million worldwide cancer cases each year, roughly 3 million are caused by poor diet, 1.5 million by infection and 1.5 million by toxins.

In fact, each cancer is as individual as you are. A cancer is almost certainly caused by a combination of factors with poor diet and/or toxins weakening the body, its cells and its immune system, laying it open to other factors like a specific carcinogen or a virus.

The truth is that almost everyone who succumbs to cancer is both nutritionally deficient **and** nutritionally toxic.

Nutritional deficiency is increasingly evident and largely due to poor eating habits coupled with a decline in the nutritional values of our foods; whether it be our tendency to fast foods or the decline in mineral content of our vegetables and fruits. Nutritional toxicity is a widespread, self-inflicted condition largely caused through consuming too much sodium and too little magnesium and potassium. Large volumes of dairy consumption can reduce magnesium absorption.

Salt may be in the form of sodium chloride (table salt) or sodium nitrite (preservative). Although the UK Food Standards Agency (FSA) argues that 6 gms of salt per day is correct for adults, in my book *The Tree of Life: The Anti-Cancer Diet*, I argue for 1 gm of sodium as a maximum and recent US Government research confirms the probable figure is 1.5 gms of sodium. By contrast the average British male consumes up to 10 gms of salt per day; in sausages, bacon, bread, baked beans, breakfast cereals, processed food, packaged foods and Chinese meals. Sodium is half the 'weight' of salt.

The Tree of Life covers this detail. Sodium and potassium are contra-balancing minerals. The power stations need potassium, and a pump on the cell surface needs magnesium to pump potassium in and sodium out. If the system falls down, the sodium displaces the potassium in all the energy producing reactions in the power stations. However, years of evolution have made those reactions demand potassium, anything else may allow the reactions to continue, but less efficiently and using less oxygen. As a result cellular oxygen levels are depressed, sodium salts abound and are more acid than the intended potassium salts. The more acid the cell is, the more inefficient the process and so a downward spiral sets in, quite possibly ending in a cancer cell.

There are more nutritional factors that can help. Nations with high nitrilosides in their diets seem not to get cancer, largely because the unique enzymes in a cancer cell turn their constituents into cyanide thus killing the host cell, whilst allowing adjacent healthy cells (which do not have the enzymes) to survive.

Or vitamin C, which apart from its antioxidant effect seems to be capable of oxidizing the internal workings of a cancer cell, and thus killing it. But then many other vitamins and minerals, loosely called antioxidants have been found to help the fight against cancer.

As we noted in the Introduction, the French have just completed a study amongst 17,000 people across seven years and using five antioxidants (vitamins C and E, beta-carotene, zinc and selenium). During that time they found that men's cancers fell 31 per cent whilst deaths from cancer fell 37 per cent during this time. Antioxidants correct deficiencies, neutralise nasty free radicals, work quickly and increase survival times. A large number of research studies provide hard evidence that they are very effective in their involvement with cancer.

Other vitamins have been shown to help defeat cancer over the last few years, often at much higher levels than the RDA. For example, antioxidant Coenzyme Q10, vitamins D and K.

Then there are supplements like fish oils, garlic and soya isoflavones that can rebalance cells and limit the formation of blood supply to tumours. These are covered extensively in *The Tree of Life* and it is not our intention to repeat them here.

But then there are wonderful immune system boosters like Essiac or Hoxsey. Or glycoproteins – these polysaccharides that help the immune system communicate with other cells and improve its ability to recognise rogue cells. Four Nobel Prizes for medicine have been won in the last ten years on these polysaccharide/protein molecules.

Diet therapies have probably never been so diverse as we learn more and more, and the overwhelming truth is that diet 'science' is merely in its infancy.

The Gerson Therapy
By far the best-known diet therapy is The Gerson Therapy. Dr Max Gerson first started to develop his theories and treatment in the 1920s for tuberculosis before emigrating from Germany to the USA in 1938. After much success, he was asked to treat someone for their cancer. After more successes, he published a book *A Cancer Therapy: Results of Fifty Cases*.

The basic principle in the Therapy is to re-stimulate the natural immune defences of the body by returning the cells to their ideal state.

This means cutting out all toxins, pesticides and herbicides by the exclusive use of organic foods, then adjusting the diet to cut out sodium, sugar, fats and protein all of which can unbalance cells, whilst increasing levels of helpful minerals, vitamins and digestive enzymes.

In practical terms the Therapy involves eating organic fruits and vegetables, whilst consuming freshly pressed organic vegetable and fruit juices every hour, thirteen times. There is a full review of the basics behind the therapy in *The Tree of Life: The Anti-Cancer Diet*.

The dramatic changes in cellular composition can result in cancer cells being flooded with 'nutrition' that they cannot abide! When the treatment works, cancer cells literally liquefy, their rogue metabolism failing.

Unfortunately this creates it's own problem. Namely, that the failing cancer cells pour their toxins out into the blood stream overloading both the blood and the liver, the organ of detoxification. This necessitates a constant cleaning and flushing of the liver. Gerson suggested using coffee enemas to encourage the liver to propel the excess toxins into the intestines.

Coffee enemas
(for more information on coffee enemas try www.enapure.com) *This piece is for information only and is not intended to be medical advice. Indeed medical authorities consider the use of coffee enemas, dangerous practice.*

How does the coffee work?
The active ingredients of coffee, when it is contained in an enema, are quickly absorbed because the veins of the anus are very close to the target tissues. The ingredients are also in a higher concentration having not been diluted in the stomach and the blood system.

The coffee works in two ways:-
First, the enzymes in coffee (palmitates) encourage the freeing of toxins held in the liver and the passing of them into the bile.

Second, active ingredients in coffee life caffeine, theobromine and theophylline dilate blood vessels and bile ducts allowing the toxic bile to pass more freely into the intestine.

How is the enema prepared?
Using organic coffee and distilled water, make the coffee normally in a cafetiere.

Leave for about an hour until lukewarm, separate the grounds and administer the equivalent of about eight cups of coffee using an enema kit that you can buy from large pharmacies.

Is that all?
Well no. The best results are apparently obtained if accompanied by a stomach massage when the lower colon is flooded.

Furthermore, other treatments may be needed to ensure the toxins from the bile are not re-absorbed into the bloodstream from the colon. Castor oil taken by mouth or enema can help removal.

In addition to the organic regime, Gerson prescribed hydrochloric acid, pepsin, pancreatin and other enzymes prepared from raw liver, together with injections of B-12, niacin and Royal Jelly supplements. As he developed his therapy he dropped the raw liver and used linseed and flaxseed oils.

He was also fastidious about unhealthy teeth and mercury filings, removing all at the start of the treatment.

The Nutritional Cancer Therapy Trust
Lawrence Plaskett, vice chair of the Nutritional Council in Britain is a fan of Dr Max Gerson and in the mid 1990's he updated the Gerson Therapy using the latest nutritional research.

He uses less juices, (favouring carrot and apple) and less coffee enemas. His University course has trained many fully qualified, expert nutritionists and, although he does not treat patients himself, such nutritionists can be contacted through The Nutritional Cancer Therapy Trust in the UK. There is undoubtedly one in your area. More explanation of the details of the Therapy are covered in *The Tree of Life*.

Other nutritional cures and diet 'therapies'
Kristine Nolfi, a Danish Doctor, adopted one of the most straightforward 'cures'. She cured her own cancer using a totally organic, vegetarian raw-food diet. She then developed the same methodology at her own 'health farm'. However, she lost her licence to practice, apparently accused of employing 'dangerous' methods!

In New Zealand an identical approach worked for **Dr Eva Hill**, whilst in South Africa **Johanna Brand**, a naturopath, cured her stomach cancer in the 1920's by eating nothing for just six weeks but organic grapes, particularly black varieties.

The Hippocrates Health Institute in Boston has branches worldwide and its founders Ann Wigmore and Victoras Kulvinskas use organic wheat grass and a vegetarian diet. Ann used this method to cure her own cancer.

Dr Johanna Budwig – This diet involved a vegetarian and raw food diet, with flaxseed and linseed supplements combined with 'quark' or German cottage cheese made from lactic acid raw skimmed milk.

The theory is that the sulphur amino acids in the quark combine with the fatty acids in flaxseed oils to restore normal cellular energy production by driving the oxygen system of healthy mitochondria. Cancer cells are thus oxidised, and reconvert to healthy cells or die.

Dr Hans Nieper – He followed much the same principles as above but added a wide range of supplements to retard and destroy tumour growth, reinforce liver function and re-strengthen the immune system.

Dr A Ferenczi – a Hungarian, used up to 1 kilogram of beetroot per day to cause tumours to breakdown. The purple of the beetroot contains anthocyanin, which has a known anti-cancer effect.

Dr Seeger, another German, uses Zell Oxygen to re-start the oxidative process in the cancer cells in an attempt to either destroy them or normalise them. Zell Oxygen is a culture of young yeast cells very high in oxygenating enzymes and works best in combination with Royal Jelly.

Macrobiotics and the Bristol Cancer Help Centre – The Macrobiotic Diet and that of the Bristol Cancer Help Centre are both covered in *The Tree of Life* and in *Everything You Need to Know to Help You Beat Cancer*. They take people back to basics. The Macrobiotic diet argues for a local, fresh and in-season diet of fruit and vegetables plus whole grains. The Bristol Cancer Help Centre largely refers people to a dairy-free, organic, vegetarian diet.

But, a word of warning. Several studies in 2003 have shown that certain cancers develop in people with low levels of vitamin B-12. B-12 is most usually found in meats. And so a vegetarian diet is deficient in B-12 (73 per cent of vegetarians are deficient in B-12). If you decide to undertake a vegetarian diet it is absolutely essential that you take good supplementation, especially B-12. (A good source is chlorella). You would also be wise to supplement your vitamin A levels too, (see chapter 14).

Mexican Clinics – There are a number of clinics and 'health centres' just across the Mexican border; some chased there by a zealous FDA in the USA, others of Mexican origin. A few have practices that may be questioned, but many submit themselves to rigorous investigation by the authorities. Whilst some might use body energy therapies or ozone therapies, others vitamin C therapy or Hydrazine Sulphate, virtually all use nutritional therapy as well, usually a form of Gerson Therapy.

There can be no doubt that **some** cancers are caused by poor diet, and that some people have most definitely used a 'good' diet to reverse this process.

There is however an important saying in the English language: 'One man's meat is another man's poison'. As our knowledge of the science of diets and human biochemistry becomes more sophisticated, so too does our appreciation that a vegetarian diet might not be right for everyone with cancer. Later in this book you will find chapters on 'metabolic typing' – read them carefully too.

3 California dreamin'

An interview with Charlotte Gerson by Chris Woollams

icon November 2003

It's a cool, clear sunny Californian winter's day and I've driven down to San Diego to meet with the famous octogenarian Charlotte Gerson, daughter and missionary of Dr Max. She of juices and coffee enemas; of health and vitality; she with no liver spots on her hands (or so I've been told).

San Diego is sunny, heavily influenced by the sea and the wide streets are clean and relatively traffic-free. I pull up outside a wooden, double-fronted building on the corner of 2nd and Cedar. This is the new home of The Gerson Institute.

I enter to meet the lovely Kristina Wylie who has a smile sunnier than the whole of California. I told her of my mission, gave her my book and six back copies of **icon** and started to ask my questions. Kristina immediately passed me onto Andrew Printer, the executive director, whilst she went off to have a chat with her roommate. Very soriety. But it's not nice to be 'dumped' however cute the smile.

Andrew welcomed me in their new building, their 'shop front' as he called it, which had made them "far more visible in the local community." They moved in eight months before. Down the road, but importantly over the border in Mexico, is The Gerson Clinic, opened under a license agreement on 1 May 2002. In California no one is allowed to treat cancer patients with anything other than the unholy trinity of surgery, radiotherapy and chemotherapy. Hence in San Diego they advise; in Mexico they treat. "It's a major step change", he adds.

Andrew started by explaining that Dr Max Gerson had developed his diet therapy and summarized it in his book *A Cancer Therapy: Results of fifty cases*. Dr Max lived from 1881–1959 and developed his theory that better health came from better nutrition.

Unfortunately the title of his book had over-focused people's views on cancer as the Gerson forté, when in reality their therapy was applicable to all diseases. Max's daughter Charlotte founded the Gerson Institute. Twenty years ago she was the rebel, fighting the orthodox medical establishment, but now The Gerson Therapy was widely accepted as THE alternative therapy, with the Institute being recognised as a leader in Alternative Medicine.

I asked about their views on other aspects of healing apart from diet, like exercise, or meditation or other complementary therapies. Andrew replied that they were looking at this right now and in the process of drawing up a wider program.

"If you believe that proper nourishment is critical, but that crops are depleted of nutrients, what are your views on supplements?" I asked. They are formulating views on that subject too.

"What does the future hold?" Andrew told me they would like to move on from their current surroundings and even open a residential "detox and spa centre", which could double as a training centre. Maybe there could be several in different locations catering to local communities.

Andrew firmly believes that after "20 years of Charlotte flying in the face of orthodox medicine", they are now established. They even advertise in the national magazine *Alternative Medicine*.

"In the past we have primarily treated people who have been given up on by orthodox medicine, people who may have just months to live. In the future we want to move to a prevention protocol, to educate the 38-year-old woman with two children that she can detox for a couple of days and do herself some good".

Andrew continues to explain that now they are more "visible", they can have more "local seminars", offer cooking classes, training and even go into local offices to offer preventative advice. Whilst they cannot treat people in California they can "direct people to our books and clinics".

Why do I get the feeling I've heard all this before? Oh yes, I remember. I spent 22 years of my life in advertising agencies! I can spot a marketing pitch at 100 paces.

Gerson have "facilities"; one in Mexico and one in Liverpool, England. "To be a facility requires a four-part, three-year training; plus we have support groups that have to come up to our standards in a three-day training programme, plus a network list of people who used our therapy with success" says Andrew.

They have lots of books and booklets for sale, plus a bi-monthly newsletter. They have membership specials, merchandise sales and class registrations at their open houses. The marketing programme unfolds and I suddenly realise even those who claim charitable status can be big businesses.

Indeed, I asked questions about The Gerson Therapy and their specific reasons, for example, for not using soya, and I was told I should subscribe to the magazine. When I asked for more details on the Therapy I was told I should buy the book. Now call me old fashioned but firstly I'd given them mine for free, and secondly I'd gone out of my way to go to San Diego to write about Gerson and give them free publicity!

I decided it was time to leave, but I would return two days later to meet Charlotte at the "Open House", a little marketing festivity taking place on Sunday afternoon. And this I did.

Charlotte is 80 years old and has more energy than most twenty-somethings. She networked the room, which contained a mixture of adoring fans and cynics, and, yes, she has no liver spots! I decided an open house required an open mind. And I must admit to being a fan of Dr Max's theories, anyway.

There was a practical demonstration of juicing: you have to have a machine that juices, and then presses to give the maximum liquid volume and mineral content. Fresh juices are essential because they are 'living' and contain enzymes as well as nutrients. By contrast Charlotte was clearly unimpressed when asked about Noni juice "it's bottled, so I don't feel it can be very good". By the way the juicer costs about £1,500, and is slightly larger than your average kitchen sink! They didn't have a practical demonstration of coffee enemas. I'd been rather looking forward to that.

I asked Charlotte about her anti-soya views. I'd read pieces she had written and the attacks were basically three-fold. Firstly, that soya milk contains ten times the aluminium level of milk; secondly, it causes allergies and, thirdly, it contains phytic acid in large quantities, which blocks mineral absorption.

I put it to Charlotte that her figures on aluminium were actually wrong. Her reply was simple: "Never mind that", and she seamlessly moved straight to allergies, citing several case histories of children. I don't doubt many things cause allergies, milk too, but individual case histories do not constitute 'proof' in my book because you rarely get simultaneous case histories for the opposition. From my own research I fully accept that soya has only been around in the West for 40 years and almost certainly milk does cause allergic reactions, but a little science would not have gone amiss. Which leaves phytic acid, which I opinioned was in many plants and all pulses not merely soy. "But in the Far East only the Japanese eat soy and that is fermented in tofu" she cried. It wasn't even worth arguing. (The Chinese make breakfast from soya milk and rice as a staple; I've been there and seen them do it. The Thais use soya – I've lived there.) When Charlotte speaks, it is hard to get anything through. She talks at you, not with you.

This is a strict, single-minded statement of a mission not to be questioned or debated. And this is the 2003 version of the mission. Changes made in previous years may have been deliberate or accidental but you will never find out.

Please don't get me wrong. I was also very impressed by her. She stands upright, drinks fresh carrot juice and talks animatedly and knowledgably. I was impressed. But then I was also impressed when Robert Maxwell spoke, so maybe I'm no one to judge!

The Therapy itself, I believe, if anything is undersold. Constant references to juicing and coffee enemas leave the science behind it ignored.

Nowadays we know that the cellular power stations, or mitochondria, normally thrive on chemical reactions involving potassium and this renders them slightly alkaline.

When the body has too much sodium it displaces the potassium, making the energy production inefficient, the mitochondria more acid and the cells toxic. They thus use less and less oxygen, produce even less energy and continue a downward spiral.

In this modern day and age there are many ways of making a cell toxic, from asbestos to oestrogen mimics, but sodium excess is how you mainly do it with your diet. A gram of sodium would be more than enough for homosapiens 3000 years ago. Nowadays the average adult American eats 16 grams per day!

It was this basic principal that Dr Max Gerson attacked over 50 years ago. Indeed he was so ahead of his time that even he did not fully understand the importance of magnesium and its ability to help pump sodium out of the cell and potassium in. Luckily the foods (nuts, apples, carrots – oh and by the way lentils, broad beans, peas, other pulses and potatoes) that are high in potassium also happen to be high in magnesium too.

I must admit I am a believer in the basic principle of the Therapy. Charlotte said simply that, "a strong and healthy immune system is capable of keeping the whole body strong and healthy. But that if the body, (and particularly the liver and the immune system), is depleted of essential nutrients, it will become sick and will not have the building blocks to heal itself."

The Therapy is a total solution, so I was told. 10–12 pounds of raw organic fruit and vegetables per day plus juices every hour freshly pressed provide the vitamins, minerals and enzymes needed to correct deficiencies. No sugar, salt and no ingested toxins. Dairy is not allowed until much later and then as no-fat cottage cheese or yogurt. Soya is never allowed, as Charlotte specifically sticks to the view that all pulses contain phytic acid and this blocks mineral absorption. But this is only the start. The patient has to detox, to clean the liver and to recharge it. After all, "preservatives, pesticides, and toxins have all inhibited its ability to function and it is the principle organ of health in the body". Clean water and juices detox, but they also cause the tumour to decompose releasing more toxins into the blood, so coffee enemas are used to clear the liver, as is the occasional dose of castor oil. Case histories talk of remarkable results from Multiple Sclerosis to breast cancer; from prostate cancer to Auto Immune Deficiency (which Charlotte is clear, doesn't really exist).

After another chat with Andrew and a longer one with Charlotte, Charlotte spoke to the eighty people previously milling around the open house. She spoke without notes for about 50 minutes. In London recently she did much the same for well over an hour. It's more like a cosy chat than a speech. But it is a dictum.

In San Diego she animatedly waved a piece of paper. She had just received a fax, she told us, a fax that informed her that the FDA, which had been under severe work pressure reviewing and approving all these (nasty) drugs had taken on more staff. Their 500 'policemen' normally employed were simply not enough to cope with all the drug applications. They had been to the US Government, but no money was forthcoming. To relieve them of their predicament, the pharmaceutical companies were to 'lend' them 750 workers. The poachers turned gamekeepers. True or not, this story certainly had her excited.

The cosy chat continued; healing anecdotes and claims. It's a chat she has clearly given a number of times. I was actually reminded a little of Tony Blair. I was hearing 'sound bites' not information, and what I found saddest was that many of the sound bites were too glib and any challenge met with a smile and little objective response. All too often the statements are almost correct, but not exactly. Try some yourself:

"Laetrile (B17) … does not cure cancer by itself. It is only used by Gerson physicians for pain relief" or "Ozone Therapy is another form of oxygen". Then there was "Jesus the vegetarian" (and I thought he was into loaves and fishes); or "Healing the incurable". Or "Gerson has had 60 years of successful treatment".

It's "nearly land", a world that talks of "relationships in the local community", of "Prevention Protocol", that describes Michael Gearin-Tosh's experiences in detail, but actually doesn't get the facts quite right, (I've read the book 'Living Proof': A Medical Mutiny, heard him speak and met him). And it's such a shame, because I so wanted to believe.

4 Eat to beat cancer?
John Boik – a total attack on cancer by natural compounds

Chris Woollams

The gremlins are out in force again. You remember the gremlins – they're the terrorists that gave that loveable Mugwai a tough time. One moment there's a calm Mugwai – a few drops of water later and he's surrounded by a thousand screaming hell raisers bent on causing the downfall of civilisation.

Well that was the story according to Spielberg.

But, it seems, gremlins are not just a figment of a film director's imagination.

Take the article printed in the British Journal of Cancer (2004, 90, 408-413). A simple story really. A team of scientists set out to find out how many patients take supplements, and which ones.

The research basically concluded that of 318 patients studied, 51.6 per cent took supplements and of these 47.6 took a mixture of supplements and herbal remedies. The report should have taken about half a page. Instead it went on for six pages and was entitled 'Potential health risks of complementary alternative medicines in cancer patients'.

The initial summary of the paper started, "Many cancer patients use complementary alternative medicines, but may not be aware of the potential risks". Not in the least bit contentious that statement then!! Firstly note that herbal remedies and supplements have now become both complementary and alternative simultaneously; add to that their classification as medicines and you can see the first drops of water hitting our Mugwai. We know what's coming don't we?

The report published a table listing some of these complementary alternative medicines (CAMs) with a column for "Approved by German regulatory authority", another for selected other/unproven (claimed effects that is), and a column for suggested mechanism of action.

The report included little gems such as:

"Unconventional cancer therapies such as Laetrile, Essiac and Coenzyme Q10 may not be effective."

"Supplements may be associated with adverse events including bleeding and liver failure." (No mention, save a reference, was made of which supplements.)

"Or fail to work, for example, high dose vitamin C (Cregan et al 1979)."

There was not one serious mention of a benefit of any herb or supplement backed by research. As readers of **icon** know, I write a monthly review of a vitamin or mineral and include numerous references to scientific papers. Yet again this BJC report quoted the "beta-carotene taken by smokers/asbestos breathers increases risk of lung cancer" research study. As readers of my review on beta-carotene will know, there have been more than twenty reviews in the last few years of the proven anti-cancer activity of beta-carotene.

Personally, I regard the piece in the *British Journal of Cancer* as hopelessly unhelpful to everybody. However, a famous 'complementary expert' disagrees and was quoted in many newspapers warning of the dangers of CAMs.

But then he has also co-produced a report on websites and has concluded that they can be very misleading; although he did approve of 'Quackwatch' from the USA. Since the advent of the National Centre for Complementary and Alternative Medicines in the USA, gremlins intent on causing subjective havoc have been driven underground – on to the net. Quackwatch is one of those; its nadir coming when it rubbished the effectiveness of acupuncture. Still, we're all entitled to our opinions.

Much more worrying is that any doctor, scientist or gremlin wishing to be thoroughly informed could have read all about every such CAM in copious detail since March 2001. It was then that John Boik launched his book, *Natural Compounds in Cancer Therapy*.

Now, John Boik knows a thing or two about such natural compounds. He is a Co-investigator of Research Projects at the MD Anderson Cancer Center at the University of Texas. We are talking top-drawer cancer centre now. And he is on the Editorial Review Board for the journal *Alternative Medicine Review*. An acupuncturist, Boik has studied everything from herbs to oriental medicine.

And this book is no ordinary book. **It contains over 4000 references to published scientific reviews.** It covers pretty well all the actions of all the natural compounds and is thoroughly referenced; it is often described as the ultimate reference guide. So, the gremlins have little excuse for bad behaviour.

He makes a number of points. For example, that misinformation abounds in health treatment and cancer, but worse is the level of **disinformation** on natural compounds.

So he has recorded hundreds of pre-clinical studies demonstrating the potential of natural compounds.

But probably his most crucial point for cancer patients is his view that it is very unlikely that there can ever be a single 'magic bullet' cancer cure. Where natural compounds are concerned, he believes you have to look for a combination of compounds, just as we would eat in nature.

The logic is simple. Cancer is not about just one event. It is about a number of changes inside a cell, cancer cell formation, rapid division, growing a blood vessel supply (angiogenesis), metastasis etc. And in nature we would eat a variety of products, some of which might help protect us against each eventuality.

He divides such natural compounds into 'direct activity' (can work directly against cancer cells), 'indirect acting' (which help to create an environment in and around cancer cells) and immune system stimulants' (affecting the quantity and quality of the immune system).

He lists forty or so compounds divided into a number of groups – the aim being to select an item from each group to help achieve a certain desired effect in the anti-cancer process.

He includes flavenoids like quercetin and genistein, curcumin, omega 3 fatty acids from fish oils, garlic, limonene resveratrol, selenium, vitamin A, vitamin D, vitamin E, grape seed extract, vitamin C, bromelain, astragalus, shiitake, ginseng, glutamine, melatonin – in fact virtually all the regulars we cover in **icon** month in, month out.

So there we have it. Natural compounds can and do target every part of the cancer process, whether it is their ability to metastase or their ability to hide from the immune system.

And if it's good enough for the MD Anderson Cancer Institute, it is certainly good enough for **icon**. So gremlins beware. We are simply not going to sit back and let you terrorise our backyard!

Cancer patients deserve to know the truth, the whole truth and nothing but the truth. And that's why we formed CANCERactive.

5 Natural Progesterone

Chris Woollams

icon September/October 2004

Progesterone – The Natural Protector
Don't be confused!
The Women's health Initiative in the USA runs from 1997 to 2005. One trial within it looked at HRT. This trial was split into two separate parts: a group of women who took oestrogen-only HRT, and a group of women who took oestrogen/progesterone-HRT. In August 2003 the latter group trial was stopped. The mixed HRT had increased breast cancer cases 100 per cent. The oestrogen-only group was allowed to continue. It had 'only' seen a 27 per cent increase. The difference between the two groups? **SYNTHETIC PROGESTERONE.**

The subgroups in the WHI study were quite small. But the research has been confirmed by a much larger study, namely Cancer Research UK's Million Women Study. Here scientists found that women using 'combination' HRT were twice as likely to develop breast cancer as non-users (In other words, again, a 100 per cent increase).

In developing countries amongst 1000 post-menopausal women who do not use HRT there will be about 20 cases of breast cancer between the ages of 50 and 60. For every 1000 women who begin 10 years of HRT at 50, those on oestrogen-only will develop about 5 extra cases, those on oestrogen-progesterone combination HRT will develop 19, or four times more cases.

Nylon versus Cotton

Now, there are some doctors who feel that synthetic progesterone is a significant cause of cancer. We receive letters from them. The indications are certainly there.

However, many people (doctors included) get completely confused between synthetic progesterone and natural progesterone. They are as different as two shirts, one made of nylon and the other of cotton.

Synthetic progesterone in fact, should not be even called progesterone. Its name in the UK is **progestagen** and in the USA, **progestin.**

Patently different

icon recently covered research showing that vitamin A had a significant effect on a cancer. The conclusion of the research was that now drugs could be made to have a real effect on the cancer. But why not use vitamin A? The answer is simple. A natural substance cannot be patented. Without a patent there is no profit for a pharmaceutical company and no incentive to recommend the treatment. Sad but true. And doctors receive most of their information from pharmaceutical companies so they never come across the original research, which lies dormant.

So too with natural progesterone; made from natural sources it cannot be patented and is thus an outcast – confined to the dustbin marked 'not a source of profit'. Meanwhile the man-made equivalents are widely used. BUT. Progestagens are synthetic hormones that are similar **but not identical to** natural progesterone. Even slight changes in hormones can, and do, cause considerable side effects in the human body.

Natural Function and cancer

Progesterone is the hormone produced by the female ovary after ovulation. However in the Western world, diet and lifestyle have made periods far more irregular and, although a woman may bleed, she may not have ovulated. Thus she may make far less actual progesterone across the average year than God intended.

One of the major evolutionary functions of natural progesterone is to balance and oppose oestrogen. After ovulation the ovaries produce approximately 20 mgs per day of progesterone, stopping any further oestrogen-induced ovulations. During pregnancy the placenta produces more than 300 mgs of progesterone per day for similar reasons. Indeed Cancer Research UK has shown that breast cancer rates fall the more children a woman has.

A 30 year retrospective study at John Hopkins University in the USA showed conclusively that women who were progesterone deficient had 5.4 times the level of breast cancer and 10 times more deaths from cancers of all types (AM. J. Epidem. 114.2 1981).

Other Benefits
Progesterone supports and maintains pregnancy. It is a precursor to a number of other hormones. It has receptor sites in bone cells, nerve sheaths and in brain cells indicating that it plays a role in all their functions. There are two or three scientific trials (e.g. Smith, Gung, Hsu – Nature 1998 and Magill P, Br.- J Gen Pract; Nov 1995) that imply it will help in PMS.

The Progesterone Problem
Menopause is not something that happens suddenly. From the age of 35 most women's progesterone levels start to decline as they gradually stop ovulating or 'splutter' out of eggs (significant levels of progesterone are only produced from the empty follicle after a women ovulates). At these times the adrenals are the sole source of the natural hormone, but only producing 3 per cent of the original amount. Indeed less progesterone than is normally produced by a man!

On the other hand, oestrogen levels can remain high right up until menopause when they will decline to approximately 40 –

60 per cent of original levels, just enough to stop ovulation, (oestrogen is also the hormone that builds up the womb lining). Thus oestrogen is still produced in quite large quantities (it is also made in muscles for example) yet progesterone is drastically reduced. Couple this with the effects of certain pesticides or toiletry ingredients, for example, which are known to mimic the action of oestrogen in the body and a woman can suddenly experience severe oestrogen dominance. And excess oestrogen is linked to an increased risk of cancer.

The balance between oestrogen and progesterone poses other questions. For example, if osteoporosis is a condition of the menopause when oestrogen declines, why are so many women with regular cycles reaching menopause with osteoporosis well underway? One counter argument is that the bone building benefits of progesterone have been severely hampered over time by the synthetic versions in the pill or other synthetic oestrogen providers.

Hot flushes can occur when the oestrogen is declining 'around the age' of menopause when a woman is having anovulatory cycles (not ovulating) and the follicle stimulating hormone is working like fury trying to squeeze any last drop of oestrogen from the ovaries.

Is the solution to increase your oestrogen further by taking HRT with all the associated risks of cancer, or is it to try to maintain the original balance by increasing natural progesterone instead?

That high levels of oestrogen are ever present in women is all too clear to scientists if not to doctors. A recent study on oestrogen confirmed that overweight post-menopausal women actually have higher oestrogen levels than thin pre-menopausal thus exploding the myth that somehow your oestrogen levels have declined dramatically! Moreover, the new aromatase inhibitor drugs have been designed to cut high oestrogen levels in post-menopausal women. Now, I thought Doctors had been dishing out HRT because post-menopausal women had so little oestrogen – silly me.

So, is oestrogen deficiency even the cause of osteoporosis? The progesterone receptor sites and bones might indicate otherwise. As we have told you before in icon, the Western world has the highest levels of blood calcium and the lowest levels of bone calcium in the world. Both are directly due to a high dairy consumption. Dairy depresses magnesium and vitamin D levels, both essential for calcium uptake into bones. One of the standard answers to osteoporosis is "consume more dairy". The real answer is clearly more complex than this and involves hormones like progesterone, and importantly actually consuming <u>less</u> dairy (a good helping of green vegetables will give you your daily calcium).

Breast cancer

Dr Paul Layman wrote to us recently to clear up an error in the Tony Howell interview. Paul writes, *"An eighteen year study on the protective effect of natural progesterone has recently been confirmed. The oestrogen receptor status of breast cancer is now thought to be of significance in recurrence rates, but the Imperial College study seemed to suggest that the timing of breast surgery was more important than receptor status".*

And he is perfectly correct. **Choosing the correct point in your monthly cycle to have a breast operation can increase your 10-year survival chances by two thirds!** Every woman and their doctor should know this fact.

The Imperial Cancer Research Fund (Cancer, 15 Nov 1999) states clearly that **"Women having breast tumours removed during the follicular phase of their cycle (that is days 3-12 when their oestrogen is high) have a 10-year survival rate of only 45 per cent, compared to a 10-year survival rate of 75 per cent for women having surgery during the luteal phase (when progesterone is high)."**

Indeed the research also showed that oestrogen receptor positive and progesterone receptor positive tumours had the highest survival rates if surgery was performed in the second half of a woman's cycle.

This work confirmed an earlier study from Guy's Hospital by Cooper, Gillett, Patel, Barnes and Fentiman in August 1999 and yet earlier work by Hrushesky et al (Lancet 1989).

Natural progesterone confers protection
A further study (Formby and Wiley, Journal Nat. Cancer Inst. June 1997) shows that natural progesterone actually inhibits growth and induces cell death in breast cancer cells by affecting p53 and Bcl-2 gene expression.

This followed work by Chang, Lee et al (Fertility and Sterility vol 63 1995) that, whilst oestradiol (the most potent oestrogen hormone) increases the number of cycling epithelial cells, natural progesterone actually decreases them.

The study further states that natural progesterone secretion suppresses oestradiol receptors in both the endometrium and breast tissue, and has an anti-oestrogen effect (just as, for example, the latest aromatase inhibitors aim to do), **but that very high concentrations of synthetic progestins can stimulate human breast cancer cells.** Which takes us back to where we started. Cotton is good, nylon certainly isn't.

And men?
The work on receptor sties for prostate cancer is nowhere near as advanced. What is known is that testosterone (converted to the dangerous DHT) and oestradiol both have to be present (Monash Cancer Centre, Australia); although, according to work by Dr Thompson (Aug 2003 – Houston, Texas), oestradiol is the driving force. Quite possibly, then, there is an important balancing role for natural progesterone in prostate cancer too.

Check it out!
Natural Progesterone is available as a cream but has to be prescribed. If, male or female, you have an oestrogen driven cancer (and this can include brain tumours, colon, melanoma, prostate, breast etc) check out the possible benefits of natural

progesterone – and make sure neither you, nor your doctor are confused between cotton and nylon.

For further information please contact the excellent Progesterone Link on 01935 474343 or at www.progesterone-link.co.uk.

6 Attack of the enzymes – the pancreas strikes back
(Beard, Kelley and Gonzalez therapies)

Chris Woollams

Dr Nicholas Gonzalez has been investigating nutritional approaches to cancer and other diseases since 1981 and has been in practice in New York since 1987. He has worked with Dr Linda Isaacs since 1985.

Uniquely the National Cancer Institute is sponsoring and monitoring a full three phase clinical trial on the clinic's work. For the test they have chosen to study one of the hardest cancers to treat, pancreatic cancer.

Cancer of the pancreas is only very rarely curable and five-year survival rates are only 4 per cent in the USA.

The $1.4 million trial is supported by the NIH's National Centre for Complementary and Alternative Medicine. NIH and NCCAM are collaborating to ensure this trial is conducted with the proper scientific rigour. Why the fuss?

Gonzalez has developed an approach to pancreatic cancer using pancreatic enzymes, which have cancer-killing properties. This work originates from Edinburgh University in the early twentieth century, and Gonzalez' interest was heightened during his period of work with William Kelley DDS, who developed a general cancer treatment and recorded it in a book called *One Answer to Cancer*.

The 5-year trial uses a nutritional therapy of supplements (from vitamins to animal glandular products), plus coffee enemas and pancreatic enzymes on 90 people with Grade II, III and IV pancreatic cancers. In the earlier tests submitted in 1993 to the NCI, Gonzalez had treated a variety of cancers in a variety of patients. The NCI felt the results were not clear-cut. So they worked on a study just with pancreatic cancer patients, and incredibly patients on the Gonzalez regime lived on average 17.5 months – **or three times longer than those taking conventional chemotherapy**.

So this is political dynamite.

Background
Dr John Beard
In 1906 a Scottish embryologist Dr John Beard proposed that pancreatic enzymes represented the body's main defence against cancer.

First he noticed that in the womb, the placenta stopped growing on the precise day that the pancreas of the foetus became active and started to secrete its own enzymes (around day 56).

Since there was no logic to a foetus needing pancreatic enzymes for digestion – nutrition is provided via the placenta in a pre-digested form – he concluded pancreatic enzymes might have another function.

Beard also noted that placental cells (trophoblast cells) looked somewhat like cancer cells and hypothesised that if pancreatic enzymes could stop placental growth maybe they could do it with cancer cells too.

He then took trypsin (a pancreatic enzyme) and injected it into mouse sarcomas noting a tumour regression in every case. At the time Beard believed the enzymes had to be injected to bypass the stomach's hydrochloric acid, but in recent years it has been demonstrated that orally digested pancreatic enzymes are, in fact, acid stable.

In fact, Beard developed what is called the 'Trophoblast Theory of Cancer'. The theory runs that some undifferentiated stem cells can be stimulated by oestrogen to form 'healing cells' in normal animals. These cells act as a normal part of the healing process in animals. The other time is in the development of the placenta.

However, at the end of their action sometimes the trophoblasts are not 'switched off', and continue to produce more and more undifferentiated cells.

In some theories the body does not then attack these through the immune system because the cells are basically cells of the host anyway. In other theories the cells protect themselves by forming a protein coat around them, preventing the immune system from recognising them. Either way, Beard believed pancreatic enzymes like trypsin or chymotrypsin could attack the cells, enabling the immune system to recognise them and neutralise them.

Foetal cancer, where the foetal pancreas has not developed properly by day 56 and so produces no enzymes, is the most malignant of all cancers.

Furthermore some cancers develop from injury or shocked tissue, believed to be a result of healing cells not fully differentiating.

In 1911 Dr Beard published *The Enzyme Therapy of Cancer*, but after his death in 1923 the theory was basically forgotten, especially with the advent of Marie Curie and her radiation work.

Dr W D Kelley
Gonzalez himself became interested in this theory when he was

at Cornell University Medical School in 1981. Gonzalez had met a Dr William Donald Kelley, a dentist, who had actually been treating cancer patients for 20 years. As part of his fourth year's work he reviewed the work of Kelley, a man much attacked by the establishment for his theories, and this turned into a formal 2-year research project. In this Gonzalez reviewed 50 of Kelley's patients initially given a poor prognosis but all of who enjoyed long term survival and cancer regression with Kelley's regime.

Gonzalez then thoroughly analysed 22 patients, all of whom had visited Kelley between 1974 and 1982 with pancreatic cancer. He interviewed those still alive, relatives of the decreased and obtained full medical records.

Despite a thorough 5-year research study, the report was met with scorn and ridicule because, of course, it showed that Kelley's nutritional and enzyme approach had delivered results far beyond those of orthodox medicine.

The Kelley approach
Kelley believed every one of us have their own personal metabolic code. His aim was to find this unique metabolism and stimulate it.

Kelley took the work of Beard and theorised that the formation of cancer was clear. **Excess female hormones were responsible for changing a stem cell into a trophoblast cell.** In simple English, this means that cancer is the growth or normal tissue, but at the wrong time and in the wrong place. It progresses because of a lack of cancer digesting enzymes in the body and Kelley believed the pancreas, through its enzymes, was the primary cancer fighter in the body. So his solution was to get pancreatic enzymes to the cancer site and inhibit the growth, but control the rate of attack, otherwise toxins would flood the body and cause problems elsewhere. Kelley's treatment was divided into five parts:

1. **Nutritional therapy** – to break down the cancer cells; megavitamins, minerals, high dose vitamin C, bioflavenoids, coenzymes, raw almonds, amino acids and raw beef formula with pancreatic enzymes.

2. **Detoxification** – to cleanse the dead cells and toxins from the body; laxative purges, Epsom salts, fasts, lemon juice, coffee enemas (for anything from three weeks to 12 months).

3. **Diet** – to rebalance the body, the cellular metabolism and the immune system; at the outset he advocated a strict vegetarian diet, but modified this as he identified different individual types. Indeed he strongly advocated 'Metabolic typing' – that your ideal diet for health needed to reflect your personal metabolic type. In all he ended up with 10 different diet types and 95 variations. All diets forbade processed foods, pesticide residues, refined foods, peanuts, milk etc. They did allow almonds, low protein grains, nuts, organic raw fruits and vegetables.

4. **Neurological stimulation** – to allow free flow of body energy, especially to cancer site; for example, using osteopaths, chiropractors or physiotherapists. (A modern equivalent might be the use of a cranial osteopath to manipulate not just the skeletal structure but also the free-flow of body energy.)

5. **Spiritual** – to lift the spirits, and call upon the universal good; Kelley urged patients to trust in God, to read The Bible and to pray.

Kelley monitored a patient's progress using his own Kelley Malignancy System. Over a 20-year period, he reputedly treated 455 patients with 26 different cancers and claimed excellent results.

In 1986, probably due to endless criticism and pressure, Kelley retired. However, Gonzalez took up the mantle in 1987.

By July 1993 the then Associate Director for Cancer Therapy at the NCI invited him to present his work. What they saw proved interesting on a number of different cancers.

Pancreatic cancer was chosen for formal trials because the prognosis is so poor and so results could be obtained more noticeably and quickly. To put it in context, at the same time as the Gonzalez preliminary trial, 126 patients were treated with the FDA approved drug gemcitabine. None lived past 19 months. On the original Gonzalez regime, despite 8 of his 11 patients starting out with Grade IV disease, 5 of the 11 survived 24 months, 2 actually surviving more than 48 months!

The Gonzalez therapy
In fact, Gonzalez treats virtually all cancers and patients with MS to chronic fatigue. Each treatment protocol is individually developed.

The therapy is complex and divided into three parts:

1 Diet
2 Aggressive supplementation (nutrients and enzymes)
3 Detoxification.

The diet therapy varies by individual and cancer, and can be vegan or can require meat two to three times per day!

The supplements may number 120–175 per day, and are again tailored to the individual, including vitamins, minerals and trace elements. The aim is to improve overall metabolic function with nutrients. Every patient also takes large quantities of freeze-dried porcine pancreatic enzymes, which Gonzalez believes provide the anti-cancer activity.

Detoxification is essential as patients do go through a healing crisis and develop flu-like symptoms. Coffee enemas are used twice per day. Coffee enemas cause symptom relief for almost all patients.

Gonzalez doesn't just want to cure people. He wants his work properly tested and FDA approved. If the tests prove positive, he then wants his work included in orthodox mainstream medicine.

An interesting postscript to Beard's theories was provided in 1995 when Professor Hernan Acevedo and his associates showed that 'the synthesis and statement of LCG is a common biochemical denomination of cancer' (*Cancer*). Acevedo found LCG present in 85 different cancers examined.

So what is LCG? When a stem cell is stimulated by oestrogen it should produce a trophoblast, according to Beard. A trophoblast in turn releases a hormone called chorionic gonado trophin (LCG). Pregnancy tests usually pick up on LCG in the blood, but a similar, although much more sensitive test could detect LCG produced by cancer cells. If such a test could be developed – a sort of super pregnancy test kit – we would have a cheap and less invasive way to detect cancer via the urine.

Interestingly, when I was speaking on my UK tour, a lady told the room that she had felt so ill she thought she might be pregnant and did a test which was positive. It was only when she went to the doctors she found she had cancer instead.

Either way, it looks as though Beard's theory over 100 years ago has great merit. So why then is not more work underway? Could it be that pancreatic enzymes are cheap, or no drugs are required? Or could it be that no one receives a Nobel Prize for work that is 100 years old? Worse, when we contacted vitamin manufacturers in the UK to see if we could buy pancreatic enzymes we were told by a leading company that their sale was banned in the UK.

7 Can one diet fit all?

Chris Woollams

Where do we start? With Peter d'Adamo and his mass-market tome *Eat Right for Your Type,* or with William Kelley and his division of his patients into twelve metabolic types?

Either way the principle is the same. Your genetic structure, your blood type and your individual biochemistry; you thrive on certain foods whilst others cause problems. You know that, I know that. But do conventional cancer therapists? Or even indeed the chorus of therapists who try to drive all of us towards a standardised no dairy, all vegetarian diet?

Bill Wolcott is a founder of Healthexcel, a company that specialises in metabolic typing. Bill was a former assistant to William Kelley and claims to have worked with over 60,000 patients, of which about 25,000 were cancer patients.

As we continually say at **icon** (Integrated Cancer and Oncology News), cancer is as individual as you are. Metabolic typing acknowledges this fact.

In one respect there is no magic formula here. A good integrative doctor in the UK like Etienne Callebout or Patrick Kingsley will go to great lengths to analyse you, your metabolism and the possible causes of your disease. If you do not know the cause, how can you really begin treatment? For if smoking 'caused' your lung cancer and you didn't quit, surely even with the best treatment in the world you would expect the cancer to return.

Bill Wolcott belongs to the 'one size doesn't fit all' school of diet therapy. He became interested in Kelley's work but not as someone with a cancer to cure. Wolcott became interested in eating the foods that were best suited to his personal biochemistry. He simply wanted to be really fit and healthy and recognised that some people thrive on high protein diets whilst others thrive on carbohydrate.

Kelley has based his early work on the equilibrium of the autonomic nervous system, which is divided into two halves: the sympathetic side basically speeds you up, while the parasympathetic side shows you down. Just as eating the right foods might positively affect one half, or balance the two, so the perfect diet would help to detoxify the organs. For the nervous system is connected to the body's organs and tissues and balance in the nervous system will allow correct supply of nutrients and the removal of toxins – and vice versa.

Wolcott developed this theory to a higher level and has nine types determining characteristics clustered into three groups – he calls them the 9 Fundamental Homeostatic Controls. (Homeostasis is the word that denotes if all things are equal and we are in a natural environment we will be completely balanced.)

His 9 controls include:

1. Autonomic system (sympathetic/parasympathetic/balanced)
2. Oxidative system (fast, slow, mixed)
3. Catabolic, anabolic
4. Electrolyte/fluids – excess or deficiency
5. Acid/Alkaline – 3 types of acidosis and 3 of alkalosis
6. Prostaglandin levels
7. Endocrine balance
8. Blood type – A, B, AB, O
9. Constitutional type

It is interesting to note that control 8 is the basis for D'Adamo's theories, and that control 9 fits in with the whole principle of Ayurveda and the three Dosha's (vata, pitta and kapha).

So how should you plan your ideal cancer busting diet?

Well if you go with John Boik's view you would take a large number of natural products, just as we did in the wild and kill off **all** aspects of the cancer process. (John Boik of the MD Anderson Cancer Center has looked at all the foods we would normally have eaten in our natural environments and draw up a list of these that have benefits against aspect of the cancer process.) If you agree that your breast cancer is not the same as the lady's next door, you can go to the Internet, where at **www.healthexcel.com** you can obtain instructions and a questionnaire to set about determining your metabolic type.

With Kelley and Wolcott's theories 'You are what you eat' now takes second place to the old maxim, 'One man's meat is another man's poison'.

8 Blood typing

Ginny Fraser

NOT MY TYPE ….

> *"I believed that no two people on the face of the earth were alike; no two people have the same fingerprints, lip prints or voice prints. No two blades of grass or snowflakes are alike. Because I felt that all people were different from one another, I did not think it was logical that they should eat the same foods. It became clear to me that since each person was housed in a special body with different strengths, weaknesses and nutritional requirements, the only way to maintain health or cure illnesses was to accommodate to that particular patient's specific needs."*

These words, spoken by American naturopathic doctor James D'Adamo, inspired his son Peter to develop and promote The Blood Type diet, which burst onto the US diet scene in the mid-nineties with an almost Atkins style following. D'Adamo's first book "Eat Right for Your Type" still features prominently in high street bookshops, and just published this year is "Cancer. Fight it with the Blood Type Diet".

Generally, cancer diets recommend a vegan / vegetarian approach. Indeed, some cancer therapies such as Gerson are based on the banishing all animal proteins. The Oxford Study on vegetarians showed that they have 40% less cancer risk than non-vegetarians. Vegetarians are PC, taking care of their health and the planet, while meat eaters are on a one-way trip to blocked arteries and high blood pressure. Or so goes the conventional wisdom.

The problem, as D'Adamo saw it, was that although some people thrived on a veggie regime, others patently did not. A bit like the way some weight-loss programs seem to work for one person and not another. His Blood Type Diet was his answer to this paradox.

It is based on the idea that the different blood types evolved at different times in Man's history and thus have different pre-dispositions in the type of food that is suited to their make-up. For example, he claims that from the early Neanderthal of c. 50,000 BC the blood group of these peoples was Type O. Their diet was that of the hunter-gatherer – roots and plants and animal prey. Even today, the most prevalent blood group is O.

As the human raced moved around the world and adapted its diet to changing conditions, a different diet provoked changes in the digestive tract and immune system to help us survive in the new environments. These changes are reflected in the development of the blood types. For example, as the human race shifted from hunter-gatherers to a more agrarian lifestyle Type A appeared – initially somewhere in Asia or the Middle East around 25,000 BC – 15,000 BC. Type A is found in its highest concentration among Western Europeans.

As the races merged and migrated from the Africa to Europe, Asia and the Americas, Type B evolved around 10,000 BC. Type B is found in high numbers in Japan, China and India. Last of all, came Type AB as migration accelerated and the As and Bs mixed, and is the "newest" of blood types.

According to D'Adamo, blood type plays a huge role in determining who gets cancer and who doesn't, also which cancer is more likely to occur in which blood group, as well as the survival rate of cancer patients. This is because blood group is integral to the strength and health of the immune system.

Our immune system detects foreign substances in the body. One way it does this is by looking for antigens, found in the cells of our bodies and most other living things. If an antigen is recognised as "self", it is welcome, but if it is found to be "non-self", it is designated an intruder and dealt with accordingly, by the white blood cells.

Your blood type carries an antigen, so when your immune system is patrolling for suspicious characters, one thing it looks for is whether a suspect in question has any similarity to your blood type antigen. All of us, except AB, carry antibodies that reject the antigens of the other blood types – which is why mismatched blood transfusions typically lead to death.

What has all this got to do with cancer? According to D'Adamo, there are a number of reasons why blood type is highly relevant. First, it is important that cells of the body stay differentiated – i.e. that a muscle cell stays a muscle cell and that a fingernail cell stays a fingernail cell. The body goes to great trouble to keep the cells differentiated, to prevent the cell anarchy that leads to cancer. Blood type antigens are closely involved in differentiation.

Another aspect is that many malignant cells develop a tumour marker called Thomsen-Friedenreich (T) antigen, which has a structural similarity to the A antigen. This is normally suppressed in a healthy cell, but becomes evident as the cell moves toward malignancy. Therefore many tumours have markers which are undetectable by those with Blood Type A and AB immune systems.

According to D'Adamo, "there is undeniable evidence that people with A or AB blood have a higher rate of cancer." However, there is also research that shows a consistent link between Type O and melanoma, and Type B with bone cancer, so Os and Bs shouldn't get too complacent!

The risk of cancer is also influenced by two other factors: secretor status and the MN blood typing system (a minor blood grouping system). If you are a "secretor" then you secrete blood type antigens into your body fluids like saliva and mucus. Around 80% of the population are secretors. The rest – the non-secretors – are generally far more likely to suffer from immune diseases, but are less likely to have cancer. The MN system also plays a minor role in that type MM has a higher risk of cancer over MN and NN types.

By now you may be reeling with information. Many of us don't know our blood group, let alone our secretor or MN status! As these are tests that are not commonly available, naturopath Tom Greenfield has a clinic in Canterbury, where he treats patients with the Blood Type Diet and also provides a mail-order lab where patients can get this information.

Where does food come in? There is a chemical reaction between your blood type antigen and the foods we eat. Minimising foods that detract from proper immune function is clearly a wise move for people with cancer. Many of these "unsuitable" foods tie up the immune system unnecessarily by interacting with your opposing blood type antibodies. This is because the proteins in food also have antigens which are similar to the blood type antigens. If you eat food that contains foreign blood type antigens that will trigger your anti-blood type antibodies and the result is the agglutination (sticking together) of cells. Agglutinins in food are called lectins, and are specific to one blood type of another. Some lectins might be damaging for one blood type, yet have little effect on another. There are some lectins, shown below, that have proved to be particularly good for different blood types.

- Peanut – A, AB
- Soy bean – A, AB
- Broad bean – all types
- Mushrooms – all types
- Amaranth – A, AB
- Snail – A, AB
- Jackfruit – all types

The second significant use of blood-type specific lectins is their ability to agglutinate malignant cells (agglutination is not what you want to have happen to your normal cells, but good news for malignant cells).

So, what should someone with cancer (or hoping to prevent it) eat? Although much more detail is available in the many D'Adamo publications, below is a summary of each type, including a short personality profile and exercise preferences with each type's "superfood" also included. It is interesting to note how the profiles compare to the origins of the blood groups described earlier.

Type O
Cancer-fighting superfoods: broad bean, oily fish, seaweed, walnut, mushroom
Eat: Red meat, fish, vegetables, fruits, green tea
Avoid: Most grains (amaranth, quinoa, spelt permitted); most dairy
Curious fact: club soda is beneficial for Os
Exercise: high-intensity, aerobic
Personality type: strong, self-reliant, daring, intuitive, optimistic

Type A
Cancer-fighting superfoods: soya foods, oily fish, snail, flax oil, peanut

Eat: Fish, vegetables, fruits, dairy in small quantities, grains
Avoid: most meat (though chicken can be eaten), potatoes
Curious fact: red wine and coffee are both permitted for As!
Exercise: regular, calming such as Hatha yoga, Tai Chi, light aerobic
Personality type: co-operative, sensitive, passionate and self-controlled

Type B

Cancer-fighting superfoods: yoghurt, cultured dairy foods, ghee, oily fish, flax oil, walnuts, vegetables, fruit
Eat: Most flesh foods, turkey, fish, dairy, grains
Avoid: Chicken, soy products
Curious fact: club soda should be avoided by Bs
Exercise: mixed aerobic and stress-reducing
Personality type: the best of the Os and As, balanced, flexible, creative

Type AB

Cancer-fighting superfoods: oily fish, snail, soy foods, cultured dairy foods, vegetables, fruit
Eat: A limited amount of flesh foods, oily fish, most dairy, olive oil,
Avoid: Chicken, beef, butter
Curious fact: ABs should avoid Worcester sauce
Exercise: mixed aerobic and calming
Personality type: spiritual, relaxed, forgiving, charismatic

Tom Greenfield has been recommending the Blood Type Diet for over seven years and has seen what he describes as "incredible" results for those willing to change their eating patterns. "The most radical results have been with those in blood group O who have previously been vegetarian," he states. "Although this doesn't match the conventional diet advice, it seems that meat doesn't create as much acid in Os as grains do. The Os seem to do better on slightly acid side." Greenfield's work also bears out D'Adamo's claim that Type A women are over-represented among breast cancer patients, and especially those with MM status, in addition to all the normal risk factors such as heredity.

Greenfield points out that the Gerson Therapy was perfectly designed for the majority of people who get cancer – the Type As. However, not quite everything fits. Michael Gearin-Tosh, author of well-know cancer autobiography, Living Proof, who was a Gerson aficionado checked out D'Adamo's work and, as an A, excluded potatoes from his regime, to good effect.

There are also a number of supplements specific to blood types, but generally seen to be useful with cancer. These include Helix Plus, which may be particularly welcomed by those blood types recommended to eat snail as it contains the snail lectin! Quercitin and Larch are also highly recommended.

While the blood type diet provides a neat and simple formula, the jury is still out about how effective it is for cancer patients. It certainly doesn't have the scientific pedigree or rigour of Metabolic Typing. Dr Patrick Kingsley, Leicestershire-based cancer specialist agrees there is "a certain logic to it", but warns against one system being right for everyone. "There are so many diets to choose from – from the Stone Age diet to the Vega-tested diets – and every one of them will be inadequate for someone." Likewise, Dr Fritz Schellander, who practices in Tunbridge Wells, has some reservations and some questions about the evidence behind some of the extensive and very specific food protocols D'Adamo recommends. "Any dietary programme has to be safe, affordable and evidence-based. While this programme meets the first two criteria, I would be interested in HOW they came about their evidence for each of the foods recommended."

A register of UK-based D'Adamo-friendly doctors is available on the website www.dadamo.com.

Tom Greenfield's lab services are available on www.nature-cure.co.uk or by calling + 44 1227 761000.

9 Metabolic typing

Ginny Fraser

icon September/October 2004

One man's meat ...
We've all heard the saying that "One man's meat is another man's poison", but two – quite distinct – disciplines for identifying our highly individualized dietary needs are showing that this is literally true. Metabolic typing and blood typing are two kinds of dietary technologies that cast a whole new light on the concept of "the ideal cancer diet."

The basic principle of Metabolic Typing is that there are some foods that are bad for everyone and we all know what they are – refined sugar, processed foods, partially hydrogenated oils – but there are also **good** foods that are **bad** for you and **bad** foods that are **good** for you.

Before you rush out for a McDonald's in exasperation at yet MORE confusion about what to eat, read on. According to the science of Metabolic Typing, the style by which your body produces and processes energy determines your Type and consequently the diet that will help you to optimum health. And it may mean that foods you previously thought were unhealthy might in fact come back on the menu (though probably not the McDonald's).

It's a system that has some rigorous science behind it and a prestigious pedigree, including Dr William Kelley, a US dentist who strongly believed that each of us has our own personal metabolic code. Through identifying this unique metabolism and with his work on pancreatic enzymes, he successfully treated cancer patients for many decades, and his work was taken up – and continued today to critical acclaim – by Dr Nicholas Gonzales.

William L. Wolcott worked as Kelley's assistant for eight years and later took the understanding of metabolism to a deeper level. Dr Harold Kristal, a former pupil of Wolcott's, is another foremost practitioner in the US, while here in the UK Dr Etienne Callebout is an enthusiastic proponent of Metabolic Typing.

The system itself is one whereby you are assessed according to the acidity or alkalinity of your blood – with the ideal level being 7.46 – mildly alkaline. The aim is to get your blood to that level, and the usual view is that most of us – especially people with cancer – are too acid (from eating meat, sugary and processed foods) and that to rectify that we should eat alkalising foods like vegetables. This system shows that this might not necessarily be the best course of action.

Wolcott's research centres on the metabolism – the sum total of all physiological and biochemical reactions that take place in the body to sustain life. He states that although hundreds of thousands of biochemical reactions take place in the body on a daily basis, they all fall under the regulation of a handful of "fundamental homeostatic controls" (FHCs). Wolcott's system recognises nine FHCs, with two having primary and specific influence on diet – the Autonomic Nervous System (ANS) and the Oxidative System (OS).

The Autonomic Nervous System
The Autonomic Nervous System has two sub-branches – the Sympathetic and the Parasympathetic – which work in opposition to each other to maintain metabolic balance and efficiency. For instance, the Sympathetic nervous system speeds up the heart rate, while the Parasympathetic slows it. They work together to achieve the proper heart rate as well as the functioning of other organs and glands, which are "switched on" by

the SNS, and "switched off" by the PNS. Some people inherit stronger organs and glands that are stimulated by the Sympathetic division, and these are known as *Sympathetic Dominant Metabolic Types*. Those with organs stronger in the Parasympathetic are known as *Parasympathetic Dominant Metabolic Types*. Those relatively balanced between the two are of the *Balanced Dominant Metabolic Type*.

The Oxidative System
The other significant control is the Oxidative System which concerns the rate at which nutrients are converted to energy in all of the body's trillions of cells.

Within this group there are *Fast Oxidisers*, who are poor at metabolising fats and overly reliant on carbohydrates for energy. These people tend to burn carbohydrates too quickly but increased amounts of certain fats and proteins help balance them and normalise their energy production. *Slow Oxidisers* also have problems with deficient energy production and do better on more carbohydrates and less fat and protein in their diets.

The nine types mentioned earlier are combinations involving the pairing of the two types and are as follows:

Sympathetic Fast	Balanced Fast	Parasympathetic Fast
Sympathetic Mixed	Balanced Mixed	Parasympathetic Mixed
Sympathetic Slow	Balanced Slow	Parasympathetic Slow

In 1983, Wolcott discovered that within each pair one FHC will be *dominant* – either Autonomic or Oxidative and the significance of this is that whichever control mechanism is dominant will dictate how nutrients behave in your body. Wolcott's principle that he coined 'The Dominance Factor' effectively explained why a diet that makes you healthy, fit and trim can make your friend unhealthy, unfit and overweight. Different foods are used to balance (amongst other things) the pH of the blood, which helps upgrade or optimise all the systems of the body. Wolcott found that foods that acidify members of one group alkalise members of the other, and vice versa. Foods lower in protein and fat and higher in carbohydrate (like most fruits and vegetables) acidify the blood of the Oxdisers, but alkalize blood of Autonomic types. Foods higher in protein and fat (e.g. meat) alkalise the blood of the Oxidisers, but acidify the blood of Autonomics.

The theory is that when a person is metabolically balanced, many disease symptoms subside, and that when you eat incorrectly for your Metabolic Type it is like putting the wrong fuel in your engine – the body simply is unable to function efficiently. This failure to meet one's genetically-based nutritional requirements for the Metabolic Type, initially produces sub-clinical symptoms such as lowered energy, aches and pains, stiffness, depression, anxiety, food reactivities, constipation, insufficient digestion, etc. But left uncorrected, these conditions can develop into full-blown degenerative diseases like cancer, diabetes, heart disease, obesity and so on.

The theory does explain why there seems to be no "perfect" diet to suit everyone. William Kelley discovered this himself when he recovered from cancer using a mainly vegetarian diet, which, when he applied to his sick wife, only served to make her sicker. When he gave her some beef broth she perked up and recovered!

What type am I?
There are various ways to determine your Metabolic Type. Wolcott's book (The Metabolic Typing Diet, Doubleday, 2000) contains 65 questions to help you identify your type, and is termed a "basic" method. Questions might relate to how you feel after having a large salad for lunch (if it satisfies then you are more likely to be a Sympathetic Slow Oxidiser), or if you are often hungry (which means you are more likely to be a Parasympathetic and Fast Oxidiser).

More in-depth analyses are available for a price (between

£75 and £490) from Wolcott's organisation, Healthexcel (**www.healthexcel.com**). These range from on-line questionnaires and advisor support through to a comprehensive program (recommended for people with cancer) which involves various physiological home tests and a hair analysis which will provide an analysis of all the nine FHCs, and contain a detailed spec of supplementation, detox and lifestyle change recommendations.

Enough of the science, what do I actually eat?
As described earlier, within each dominance system (Oxidisers and Autonomics) there is both an acid and an alkaline blood type. So there are two acid blood types – the Fast Oxidiser and the Sympathetic – and two alkaline blood types – the Slow Oxidiser and the Parasympathetic. But here comes the tricky bit. Instead of putting the acid types on one diet and the alkaline types on another, the way it works out is that the acid member of one dominance system shares the same diet with the alkaline member of the other dominance system.

Let's take some common, generally considered healthy, foods to demonstrate the principle, the tomato and spinach. The tomato acidifies the Oxidisers. This is good news for Slow Oxidiser this would be help with her over-alkalinity, but it wouldn't help the Fast Oxidiser's already acid blood and would tend to exacerbate her condition. For the Automonics, then, the opposite is true – the tomato is alkalising. Good news for the Sympathetic (who runs on the acid side) but bad for the Parasympathetic (alkaline).

Spinach, on the other hand is alkalising for the Oxidisers, so for the Slow Oxidiser (over-alkaline) it is undesirable, while doing a power of good to the Fast Oxidiser. The reverse is true for the Autonomic Group – spinach is acidifying. Therefore good news for the Ps and bad for the Ss.

Are you still with me? If the whole thing makes no sense – don't worry. Take a look at what the two food groups involve.

In a nutshell, Slow Oxidiser / Sympathetic foods are lower in protein and fats and higher in complex carbohydrates. Fast Oxidiser / Parasympathetic foods are higher in protein and fats and lower in complex carbs. It's a logical system. The sluggish metabolism of the Slow Oxidiser is further slowed down by too much protein and fat, but does well on complex carbohydrates (whole grains, fruit and vegetables), which provide the quick-burning fuel they need. The Sympathetics, on the other hand, are running on nervous energy and too much protein and fat over-rev the engine of their already hyper metabolism, so their energy production is slowed down and balanced by the complex carbs.

According to Harold Kristal, another researcher in this field, what he calls "Group I"(for the Slow Oxidiser / Sympathetic) contain all grains, but states that wheat is the best of all – quite a controversial view in the light of the general consensus about wheat and its high allergy-promoting quality. Only in cases of gluten allergy should Group I types avoid wheat which has an insulin-like effect which helps Slow Oxidisers who tend to run higher blood sugar. Group Is can eat flesh proteins but only poultry and – another surprise – lean pork. As the diet is substantially lower in fats that the Group II (Fast Oxidiser / Parasympathetic) diet dairy should be limited and low or non-fat.

Group II types get what used to be the "politically incorrect" diet, until Atkins invaded the public consciousness with his high protein / high fat approach. Fast Oxidisers burn up carbohydrates too rapidly, and thus need higher protein and fat proportionately to normalize energy production. Parasympathetics tend to have somewhat sluggish systems that are worsened by the high potassium content of a high carb diet. The high protein intake in Group II foods diet will help move them into a greater balance by stimulating the weaker Sympathetic system.

Group II people should eat plenty of dark meat such as beef, lamb and liver; they can chow down on dairy (though not as a primary source of protein), but must avoid wheat and potatoes. It is important that Group IIs don't eat carbs on their own, but always have protein and fat with a meal. Whilst protein foods are pretty unlimited for the Group IIs, their fruit and vegetable menu does have some restrictions, such as the nightshade family of potatoes, tomatoes, aubergine and peppers, and cruciferous vegetables like cabbage and broccoli. Fruits should be restricted to the less sweet varieties, like Granny Smith apples.

In terms of cancer, this approach raises some interesting questions and probably confuses the heck out of many readers. "Hang on", you might be saying, "In *The Tree of Life* Chris Woollams says that vegetarians have 40% less cancer" or, "Surely the Gerson therapy advocates a totally vegetarian diet?" and "What if I am a Fast Oxidiser / Parasympathetic, am I supposed to ignore all that?" Well, other statistics may put the vegetarian issue into perspective. As Woollams goes on to say, vegetarians smoke 80% less, drink 60% less and are 80% less likely to be overweight, so perhaps their avoidance of cancer is down to those factors as much as diet.

Wolcott's point of view is, "The immune system is highly dependent for its efficiency on the "proper biochemical balance. Given the different genetically-based requirements for nutrition seen reflected in indigenous cultures all over the world, and given the clinical successes of metabolic typing over the past 25 years, it is not hard to understand that different people need different diets and different nutrient balances to optimise the immune system." He goes on to say, "If vegetarianism is so key, how can it be that cancer in the Eskimo culture where they eat 10 pounds of meat a day, huge amounts of fat, and NO CARBOHYDRATE, cancer is so rare that they did not even have a word for it in their language?!!"

What this debate highlights is that diet is a crucial area for anyone healing their cancer where they need to do their own research rather than rely on anecdotal information and received wisdom. Tiresome though it is, continuing to check out new or different information seems to be part of the package for those intent on recovery.

10 "There are no rules" – keeping an open mind

An interview with Dr Etienne Callebout by Ginny Fraser

icon March/April 2004

Doctor of Integrative Medicine, Etienne Callebout, has been described as someone with "a brain the size of a small planet", and his physical appearance – large, intense and untidy – certainly gives the impression of someone brilliant but not very concerned with the practicalities of life. Dr Callebout is one of four of the best-known 'alternative' cancer specialists who appear in the listings in the back of cancer books (along with Julian Kenyon, Fritz Schellander and Patrick Kingsley).

Belgian by birth, he has lived in the UK for some time and practices from an office in Harley Street. He is a strong believer in using naturopathic medicine to complement orthodox treatment, and often cancer patients come to him when all other options have been exhausted. He is often a last resort, and because of that his regimes – combinations of diet, supplementation, detox practices, and intravenous medication – are known to be rigorous.

He trained as a medical doctor in Belgium, but due to serious illness at the age of 19 that was cured by naturopathic medicine, he became interested in finding out as much as possible about this field. This seems to be a key element of how Dr Callebout works. He is a seeker by nature, with an intense curiosity to learn as much as possible about the many different aspects of health creation and disease. During the two hours of our interview his conversation was littered with the names of well-known researchers and scientists like Prigogyne and Klinghardt as well as spiritual teachers such as Krishnamurti, Nisargadatta and Barry Long. His CV is impressive, with qualifications in acupuncture, homeopathy, naturopathy, craniosacral therapy, and many more less mainstream approaches.

Following his qualification as a doctor, he specialised in emergency and tropical medicine, practicing in Bangladesh and Rancai (in Bihar State), where he also took time to explore places of retreat and meditation and the spiritual element human existence.

A spell of long-distance commuting followed, with a period working in both Belgium and England during the eighties, including a time as a general practitioner in Belgium and study at London's Royal Homeopathic Hospital. This was combined with working at the Letchworth Centre in Hertfordshire, a charity with a clinic attached, where he worked as a naturopathic doctor. Before moving to England full-time, he also co-founded 'Arnica' – a team of 24-hour emergency doctors who did house calls in Brussels using acupuncture, homeopathy and other naturopathic approaches, relying on this as much as possible rather than using drugs.

His move to the UK was to work full-time at the Letchworth Centre. And in 1989 his interest in cancer began in earnest, when his father died of pancreatic cancer – from diagnosis to death in six weeks. This was a great shock, and spurred him into seeking out the most up-to-date information on alternative approaches to cancer. Funding himself, he travelled to the USA and Canada, checking out as many practitioners and naturopathic remedy manufacturers as possible. "It is very important to me to be independent," he said. "The nutritional companies are no different from the pharmaceutical companies in that it is human nature to want to push their products. I wanted to check each product out myself, so that I could make the best independent choices for my patients, and change without hesitation if a better product came on the market."

"In those days, in the early nineties, this kind of medicine was quite underground, it was easier to access these people and my tactic was basically to share whatever information I had with them, which would encourage them to be very open with me. The more I travelled, the more this great exchange of information began to take place. I acquired a sense of experience and knowledge that would be difficult to get any other way. I met everyone – naturopathic doctors specialising in cancer across the USA including people like Jimmy Chan, Jesse Stoff and others. And also the people who developed metabolic typing, Harold Crystal and William Wolcott (whose books I contributed to)."

His quest for information also took him to Germany and Switzerland, which is well known for its specialist cancer clinics. He visited many of them.

Callebout is an unusual combination of the fiercely scientific and the psycho-spiritual. Trained in Psychosynthesis, he considers the philosophy of healing as deeply as the biochemistry. "I am challenging myself and the dogma that physical healing should be pursued no matter what. None of us knows what is for the highest good, so in that context I just do what I do to the best of my ability."

"The question is: How can we have a more integrative kind of therapy that brings together the emotional and the physical? It is a challenge. With cancer you have to be so focused on the biochemistry, you almost need three brains to cope with what we know and to keep abreast of it all. There is a danger of becoming so busy with the body that we lose track of the emotional side of things, for instance, what people really want."

In his practice he has learnt that the patient's own attitude to their healing is crucial. "Often people's relatives ring up on their behalf, desperate to get help for their loved one. Yet if the patient is not fully participating in their treatment and their recovery, I have learnt from experience it just doesn't work. There is a certain kind of determination that is required."

"I really only want to see people who know that I know a lot, but that I do not have the whole truth, and who also really want to help themselves in an active way. These are people who want to have an active participation in their healing and make choices. They want to be informed and are happy to challenge, not for the sake of challenging, but because they want to understand something. I also have a service that I offer for free, whereby people can call me and I will talk to them for ten minutes. If they want to take it further then they can make an appointment to come and see me."

"Nobody has the full truth about cancer, but basically what I do is try to make the body cancer-unfriendly at the same time as attacking the cancer directly. I look at all the elements that enhance cancer, and through a whole range of blood and urine tests try to check out what it is in the body that we should correct and what we should leave be. It is important that we should not annoy the person with too many elements, which is something I have done in the past."

There is no static 'Callebout' programme – it all depends on the results of the blood tests, which give information not touched upon in regular hospital blood tests. Data can be gleaned about aspects such as cell-mediated immunity, NK (Natural Killer) cells, status of the immune system and T-lymphocytes. Also revealed is whether the cancer has the ability to attract blood vessels to itself through the process of angiogenesis; whether it is secreting enzymes that eat away the immediate environment (MMP2); the capacity for apoptosis (ability of a cell to commit suicide, something cancer cells do not do naturally); gene mutation; non-genomic RNA and DNA – what is in the bloodstream that is not you – such as the fungal, bacterial and viral load.

"Not that these are necessarily carcinogenic" says Callebout, "but they keep the body busy, so it cannot deal so well with the cancer." The presence of heavy metals can also be identified. "According to English law you can't store mercury anywhere in your house, but you can store it in your mouth!" According to Dr Callebout, "There are 5–6,000 papers claiming that mercury is bad for the human system, and around 10 that say it is good! And they are based on two papers which say it is OK because 'we have always done it so'."

"Of great importance, too, are xeno-oestrogens, which have increased enormously in the last twenty years due to a combination of pesticides and pollution. These oestrogen mimicking substances can be analysed in the tissues and blood."

The way Dr Callebout works is that he combines the results of these in-depth tests with his vast experience of other experts in the field of cancer treatment. For example, he is a great admirer of the work of Max Gerson, founder of the well-known Gerson Therapy. Gerson was a pioneer of the work on sodium-potassium exchange and also introduced the use of the coffee enema as a vital aid to detoxification. "Gerson did excellent, innovative work, but it cannot be used the way he designed it," claims Callebout. "The soil is so depleted now that the vegetables simply do not have the nutritional content they had when he was working half a century ago. We also have to adapt detoxification methods to the climate. It is nice to have juices in California but can you do it in Aberdeen? You also have to take into account what people are *willing* to do. I am very enthusiastic about a soy-based product grown wild in Mongolia in specially enriched soil. But people just wouldn't take it because it tasted so bad! So I quite often had to back off on that one!"

Another area that he has subjected to in-depth scrutiny is the whole area of alkalinity-acidity – a hot topic in naturopathic cancer treatment. The conventional wisdom is that if you have cancer, then you need to keep your body alkaline. (People with cancer usually have a very acid pH.) However, important work done on metabolic typing (pioneered by Drs Kelley and Gonzalez in the USA) shows that, based on blood tests, some people acidified with vegetables and alkalised with meat – quite the opposite of the expected reaction. Cancer cells can be killed by over-alkalising and also by over-acidification (which happens during hyperthermia).

"It seems that there is a general rule that patients with the not-solid cancers like the lymphomas, leukaemias, melanomas and sarcomas do well on a high-protein, high-fat low-carbohydrate diet of a particular nature and ideally organic. All the solid cancers like breast, colon and prostate conform to the idea that a vegan diet is generally best. "

"Blanket rules are not what I do", he explained, "The more I look, the more I see there are no rules! The more I know, the more I realise I still don't know. But it is a knowledgeable "I don't know!" His attitude makes a refreshing change from the commonly-experience stance of "the doctor knows best".

"What I would say that with whatever diet is chosen, it has to be as close as possible to nature – fruitcakes do not grow on trees, and processed food takes too much effort to process. There is also a burden on the system with very cold food straight from the fridge. For some people a macrobiotic diet works very well. Then again for someone with well-advanced cancer who cannot digest food very well, raw foods (which are high in nutrients) would be too difficult for them, but cooked macrobiotic food would be good."

Dr Callebout's philosophy is simple. "Look at what went wrong, try to correct it and give an extra little push to the body. If you only aim for homeostasis then you might not get the desired effect." He quotes the work of Nobel Prize winner, Dr Prigogyne, of the Free University of Brussels, who did extensive work on this subject, who said that in order to create negative entropy i.e. evolution to a higher state, you first had to create an unstable situation in the body. "Thus, it is possible to over-acidify, over-alkalise or over-oxygenate to create a positive result."

His treatments are often tailored to work in conjunction with other therapies such as chemotherapy and radiotherapy, and he also offers supplements to limit the side effects of these treatments, plus guidance on which supplements to *avoid* in case they protect the cancer cells. He is increasingly working in co-operation with the medical establishment and often gets referrals through oncologists in mainstream medicine.

Although Dr Callebout is now a well-know alternative cancer specialist, he continues to pursue his quest for knowledge on this disease with, for instance, quarterly trips to the conferences of the American Association of Environmental Medicine. The importance of being willing to let go of one approach, and adapt and change as new information comes forward is paramount for him. He translates the old adage of "Don't live your life according to others' opinions" to "Don't live your life according to your own opinions, because they might be inaccurate, based on out-of-date information and beliefs and mainly on survival instincts."

If you are looking for a doctor with a fantastic filing system, a team of secretaries who immediately return your calls, who provides neat word-processed prescriptions, then Dr Callebout is not your man. On the other hand, if you are looking for someone with enormous eclectic experience who will treat you as an individual and not a 'cancer patient', this unconventional Belgian might be just the ticket.

11 B-17: 'Nature's chemotherapy'

Chris Woollams

icon May 2003

Natural foods

B-17 or amygdalin is a naturally occurring vitamin. In fact it is slightly wrong to think of it as a single product like, say, vitamin C. There is a group of approximately 14 products that are water-soluble, and found naturally in over 1,200 species of plant in the world. Every area of the world supporting vegetation has such plants.

The active ingredients are often described as nitrilosides or beta-cyanogenetic glucosides and there are at least 800 foods common in worldwide diets that are nitrilosidic.

Nitrilosidic foods include:

- alfalfa sprouts, bamboo shoots, mung bean sprouts;
- barley, buckwheat, maize, millet;
- blackberries, currants, cassava, cranberries, gooseberries, loganberries, quince, raspberries, strawberries, yams;
- brown rice, fava beans, lentils and many pulses like kidney beans, lima beans and field beans;
- flax seed, linseed;
- pecans, macadamia nuts, cashews, walnuts;
- watercress, sweet potato;
- almonds and the seeds of lemons, limes, cherries, apples, apricots, prunes, plums and pears.

In fact all the foods we don't eat too much of these days!!

The consumption of barley, buckwheat and millet have given way to refined wheats, and pulses like lentils which accounted for 30 per cent of our protein in 1900 now account for only 2 per cent.

Primitive tribes around the world still base their diets around B-17 rich foods. Cassava, papaya, yam, sweet potato in the tropics; unrefined rice in the Far East; seeds and nuts in the Himalayas; the salmon-berry eaten by Eskimos, or the arrow-grass of the arctic tundra feeding the caribou.

Nutritionist and scientists alike studied the various tribes. Sir Robert McCarrison in the 1920s and John Dark MD twenty years later failed to find a single case of cancer amongst the Hunzas, the tribes of West Pakistan. V Steffanson found the same with the Eskimos and wrote *Cancer: Disease of Civilisation* as a result. Dr M Navarro of Santo Thomas, University of Manilla, noticed the same with the Philippine population who ate cassava, wild rice, wild beans, berries and fruits of all kinds. Dr Albert Schweitzer noted the same in Gabon "this absence of cancer seemed to be due to the difference of nutrition in the natives compared to the Europeans." Their diet was centred around sorghum, cassava, millet and maize.

Studies of the consumption of B-17 varied from Dark's finding that the Hunzas consumed at least 150–250mgs per day, to Dean Burk, head of cytochemistry department of the National Cancer Institute in the USA in the seventies writing that the Modoc Indians in North America consumed over 8,000 mgs per day! (Dean Burke actually gave amygdalin the name B-17.)

We leave these foods aside at our peril. The World Health Organisation has, after all, confirmed that in their view a large percentage of all cancers could be prevented by simple changes in diet.

Cancer treatments
Amygdalin was first isolated in 1830 and used as an anti-cancer

agent in Russia as early as 1845. But it was reborn by the father/son team Ernst Krebs senior and junior who isolated a purified form of the active ingredient (calling it laetrile) and, with others in the late fifties to seventies, sought to explain its action.

Cancer cells differ in a number of ways from normal cells. One difference in that the mitochondria, or power stations, do not use oxygen to produce energy, and have a whole different energy production system and different set of helper chemicals (enzymes). In a cancer cell, an enzyme called glucosidase breaks down B-17 into hydrogen cyanide (which kills it) and benzaldehyde, (an analgesic). In normal cells where glucosidase is virtually non-existent another enzyme, rhodenase, renders the B-17 harmless, converting it to thiocyanate, a substance which helps the body regulate blood pressure and vitamin B-12. So, the proponents argue, B-17 is a seek and destroy missile.

Well, maybe. Every day you produce several hundred cancer cells. Get them early with a high B-17 diet and this could be true. However, as cancers develop they often form protective protein coats around the cells to ward off the immune system.

Various cancer clinics have thus developed 'therapy packages'; these include bromelain (from pineapple), papain (from papaya) and two pancreatic enzymes trypsin and chymotrypsin to break down this protein coat, plus vitamins A, E and B complex, plus high dose vitamin C and high dose minerals.

The critics say that there are no studies showing it works. This is not true.

Laetrile has shown effectiveness against cancer cells *in vitro*, and in rats and mice. Even the NCI, which is negative about laetrile, reports that by the late seventies over 70,000 cancer patients had been treated with laetrile and there are copious case histories on its effectiveness.

Krebs himself presented results on their work with cancer patients to a Congressional hearing; but since, there has been no equivalent of 'the clinical trial'. It doesn't help, of course, when the cancer authorities join forces to hound such therapies out of America. This just creates a disservice to patients who would really like to know the truth, one way or the other!

Another product of the enzyme action on amygdalin in a cancer cell is benzaldehyde. Although this can act against cancer cells both killing them and turning them into 'normal' cells (Ralph Moss: *The Cancer Therapy*) its other action is as an analgesic. B-17 can and does have a general calming and palliative action on cancer patients.

Krebs recommended eating ten apricot seeds per day for life (the seeds and kernels have the highest levels of B-17); cancer treatments use four to six 500mg tablets per day or intravenous injections.

One issue is overdosing. A maximum of five kernels at any one time is recommended for preventers, and cancer treatments have to be properly supervised. Excess B-17 and cyanide by-products have been known to build up in the liver. Each of us has different capacities and the cancer patient has an already impaired liver. Cyanide poisoning can result if excess is consumed. 1gm is the maximum recommended to be taken at any one time and the US Nutrition Almanac recommends a maximum of 35 seeds per day.

Another problem is effective dosage. In the experiments with mice and rats the dosage levels were high at 500 mgs per kilogram of body weight, and intravenous infusion was used.

The clinics that use it do use it intravenously with all manner of support e.g. supplements, diet therapies, pancreatic enzymes, oxygen therapies and vitamin C megadoses. Thus it is hard to say that B-17 alone works or exactly what combination of ingredients was necessary to get optimum results.

The general feeling is that the 'package' does work against cancer cells, especially the 'free' ones roaming the body that might start secondaries.

But feeling is not the same as a clinical trial. And anyway, should such research be conducted with just B-17 or the whole metabolic package?

Having read the original research on B-17 treatments we, at **icon**, we find the 'evidence' against laetrile almost non-existent, whilst there are overwhelming although varied claims for its effectiveness. The usual over-simplistic criticism is that B-17 contains 'cyanide' and so is dangerous. But then in the same way so does the vitamin B-12 molecule, and that is known to be absolutely essential to our health.

Yet in June 2004 UK authorities decided to outlaw the prescribing of B-17 by doctors. They cannot even obtain supplies for you. Most users now go direct to The Oasis of Hope in Mexico for supplies (see next chapter).

We simply do not understand the logic of a Government Health Authority, the FDA, concluding that it doesn't work and so moving to ban the interstate shipments of apricot kernels and planting of bitter almond trees! Even my mother's Asda 'iced log' (a cake) contained 11 per cent apricot kernel paste! Presumably this cannot be moved between California and Nevada!

And to the major UK Charity who claims on its website that 'if laetrile worked, surely it would have been developed by a pharmaceutical company by now', we say this is an appallingly poor piece of patient support. And to be as cynical as the charity in question, why would a pharmaceutical company invest millions in B-17 when it cannot be patented, and if shown to be effective would remove the market for their other products?!

12 Mexican wave

An interview with Dr Francisco Contreras by Chris Woollams

icon August 2003

Francisco Contreras loves Renaissance art, music and riding motorbikes. He has just written a book about Italy and is in the midst of his cancer tour, he intends to take three days off, and is having his leathers shipped over from Mexico so he can take a motorbike up into the Alps.

Francisco Contreras is also passionate about helping people with cancer. He truly feels he has a calling and is devoutly Christian.

His hospital, The Oasis of Hope, is a world-class facility and people come from all over the world to be treated – last Christmas people from nineteen different nations were sitting down to lunch together.

The hospital caters for all disciplines with the exception of neonatal and when I was in California I heard radio commercials inviting the ill to attend. But the reputation of Contreras and The Oasis of Hope is resolutely based around cancer treatment.

The great majority of patients arriving in Mexico have grade 4 cancers, about as bad as you can get. Contreras believes one of the first challenges is changing cancer patient's expectations of cure. "Doctors have sold people on the goal of getting rid of the cancer 100 per cent and this expectation is completely unrealistic. If they take a picture after the treatment and the cancer is still there then there is gloom, the treatment has failed", he opinions. In his view, "Living with the cancer, enjoying life anyway, being alive 5 years later, is success. It's like a good marriage. You don't bother me and I don't bother you", he laughs. In his view, happiness with your life and your cancer is linked to your expectations.

Three levels of treatment
Happiness is an important cancer-fighting emotion at The Oasis. Indeed Contreras defines his treatment programme as providing the patient with 3 resources: emotional, spiritual and physical. Of the three he immediately jumps to talk about the second.

"People who do well with us often have 'spiritual fortitude' – their view on life is so different. If you view your life just a little part of eternity, the fear factor of cancer becomes a secondary problem. We acknowledge all faiths and beliefs but we don't hide the fact that we are Christians. We believe your ticket to eternity in heaven is Jesus Christ and we counsel patients in the teachings of the Bible. We have two people in a patient's room praying for the patients and we have daily participation meetings".

In fact the walls are covered with scripture, there is a chaplin and live-in missionaries at The Oasis of Hope.

Emotional well-being is also tended to. Contreras tells the story of a lady who arrived with a bad case of breast cancer. At The Oasis of Hope they encourage partners to attend too; even to sleep with the patient in the all-private hospital. So at the preliminary meeting, Contreras was interviewing the patient with her husband in attendance. Or at least trying to! Every time he asked her a question, the husband answered! In the end he kicked the husband out of the room and, seemingly for the first time in her life she was free to talk – free to get things "off her chest". Contreras recommended counselling, she met with a counsellor every day for two weeks and left a new woman with her cancer in regression. He didn't say what happened to her husband!

Other aspects of emotional well-being are attended to, from laughter – "laughing stimulates the immune system better than any drug" – to music and even the colour of the hospital room. They organise meetings with jokes, and 'sing-alongs' at The Oasis of Hope.

We talked about research from an American Hospital that people who were more argumentative survived longer. "We are very clear. People who are more determined, beat it", he says.

Of course, it is the third level of treatment that excites him most; the physical – but more of that later.

A little history
The origins of the hospital concern a lady called Cecile Hoffman. Francisco's father Ernesto had started a free clinic for the poor called The Good Samaritan after time as a doctor in the Mexican military, and his mother had become a nurse there. Cecile had cancer and turned up in Mexico requesting that Ernesto administer laetrile to her. She had obtained supplies in Canada, but found no American hospital would use it for her benefit. And so a link to cancer and laetrile was founded.

Francisco grew up around all this. Often he would have to give up his bed as the clinic over the road overflowed. He thought about training in music but the call of medicine was too strong. After medical schools in Taluca, Mexico City and Pasedena, California he spent 5 years studying surgical oncology in Vienna.

Meanwhile the Mexican Authorities had shut the laetrile clinic and Ernesto had opened a new hospital called Del Mar, in its place. Francisco started there but wanted a world-class facility and in 1984 the all new, state of the art Hospital Ernesto Contreras opened in its place.

Building the patient relationship
Ernesto taught Francisco, especially reminding him of the roots

and reasons for their mission. Their practice has two fundamental principles:

- Do no harm
- Treat the patient as yourself.

No therapy was off-limits as long as it was potentially effective and covered the two points above. Such 'open-mindedness' is the essence and the point of difference in The Oasis of Hope, but of course it brings its critics.

Since treatments are planned individually they may include laetrile or ozone therapy, bringing criticism from official medical authorities in the USA; and they may include radiotherapy or chemotherapy, bringing criticism from alternative, natural practitioners. As Francisco himself says, "Of course, chemotherapy is a valid option and we do use it sometimes. But we just don't necessarily find it that effective!" I spoke with other Mexican clinics that indeed described the hospital bizarrely as 'too orthodox'!

In 1996 at the suggestion of a patient, the hospital's name was changed to The Oasis of Hope, and in 1997 Ernesto handed over the reins to Francisco completely.

Although they treat all manner of patients, cancer remains the focus and patient relationship the emphasis.

A course of 'treatment' typically takes around three weeks and the hospital has roughly 180 private rooms. A stay can cost between $US 15,000 and $US 20,000. But Francisco emphasises that treatment is a two-year programme, the first three weeks at The Oasis are more about education and training to enable the patient to continue the programme effectively when they return home.

Francisco emphasises that what gives him most pleasure is turning a **victim** into a **victor**; watching the successes with patients, but not necessarily total 'cures', and building a rapport and a real trust with the patient over what they are doing.

He gets disappointed a little by the FDA and the Mexican FDA 'hovering' all the time in the background, but says they have survived some heavy-duty inspections with flying colours, so even that doesn't concern him so much these days. His biggest disappointment is that there have been so very few advances made with children's cancer across the world.

The physical treatments
The patient relationship comes to the fore from the very start. He is a great admirer of Dr Gerson and their diet programme is based on the Gerson Therapy; indeed Charlotte Gerson's clinic was inside The Oasis until recently when she set up her own facility also in Mexico. (The space has now been taken by Dr Josef Issels' widow, Marie Issels another famous name in Cancer Treatment. Issels started his highly successful integrated cancer practice in 1951.)

At The Oasis they have found that success or failure with the Gerson Therapy can depend a lot on the patient's individual personality. Some patients simply find it too arduous and drop out, so The Oasis has modified it to where it is practical for most people.

There's less juicing, just four to five rather than thirteen. It is less strict, with only one or two coffee enemas not five. As Francisco says, "You've got to have time to enjoy not having cancer!" But he believes diet plays not just a physical, but a mental role too. "If you smoke, you are telling your body something; you don't care about it. If every time you eat you are making a sacrifice you are also supplying a message that you care about your body".

Every patient receives nutritional counselling. The Oasis will use drips, EDTA, polarising solutions, juice fasts, colonic irrigation and coffee enemas coupled with an essentially vegetarian diet, although recently fish has been added in.

To this detoxification programme they add vitamins and supplements often also via drips.

This is then the core of the programme, which also usually involves B-17. "We see B-17 as nature's chemotherapy. It is a wonderful supporting agent for our treatments; we usually combine it with other specific treatments and there is usually synergy. It doesn't work on all cancers; with sarcomas, primary brain tumours and primary liver tumours we have not had good results, but we still use it because it is a strong supporting agent".

They use shark cartilage in much the same way to stop tumour spread. When I referred to the early work with shark cartilage and the emphasis that bottled mass-produced products were reported near useless, Contreras told me that they always carefully prepared their own from scratch.

Treatment is very thorough at The Oasis. You are expected to arrive with all your laboratory reports and medical history, which they will review to see if previous doctors have missed anything. Then they do all the laboratory work again as a comparison.

So what else do they use at The Oasis – and what treatments excite him?

"**Ozone** is our project. It is really most exciting and we are getting real results with it", says Contreras. To date they have treated almost 1500 patients and use a machine similar to a dialysis machine to ozonate the whole blood system, (*Ed. Since 75 per cent of the blood in the body is in the poorly oxygenated venous system, the historical problem has always been how to create oxygen overload around the tumour*). Contreras also increased the PO_2 pressure from 100 to 700.

The ozone breaks down into oxygen and hydrogen peroxide, the latter enhancing nitrous oxide levels and actually helping deliver oxygenated haemoglobin past the tumour's defence systems.

(Tumours restrict the capillaries feeding them, so oxygen – which kills them – can't pass into the tumour. Nitrous oxide dilates the blood vessels.)

A second benefit Contreras says of ozone therapy is that it increases natural cytokines in the body giving a huge boost to the immune system. Contreras claims that 40 per cent of patients see tumour regression of 10 to 30 per cent within 15 days.

Contreras is always on the look out for new and potentially effective treatments. He is particularly keen to explore the latest developments in China and Russia. One Chinese project, **CHML,** makes him extremely excited. CHML involves using polypeptides taken from the lipid membranes of animal or plant cells. These polypeptides seem to act as extremely fast and effective antioxidating agents on tumours providing the delivery system can take them into the tumour. CHML must therefore be injected directly into the tumour, or provided via a catheter into the tumour's blood supply, otherwise it doesn't work. This requires phenomenal accuracy and direct access to the tumour.

The Chinese continue to develop these potent polypeptides but the FDA wants exclusive rights to develop the project outside China. According to Contreras the FDA logic for any treatment is simple. It can be miraculously effective, but it will not get approval if the FDA doesn't know how it works. In the case of CHML the FDA knows exactly how it works and wants exclusive usage. Sadly, for this reason, he may not be able to obtain and use it in Mexico.

By contrast **Photodynamic Therapy** (PDT) doesn't seem to interest him. They tried it, had lights everywhere but couldn't make it work, he claims. In fact, as readers of **icon** know, your intrepid reporter has investigated PDT quite extensively and was surprisingly unconvinced that Contreras knew what he was talking about on PDT(!). Never mind.

So what does the future bring? Contreras feels the most exciting area long term is Electromagnetic Fields, just as we do at **icon**.

MRI scanning already uses the basic principles that different tissues resonate at different frequencies and so sonographic waves can be reflected to create pictures of the tissues and any cancer cells. "If we could learn the exact resonance of cancer cells then we could destroy them whilst leaving the surrounding tissues unaffected", says Contreras. In the past a chap called Dr Royal Rife – yes, really – discovered that cancer cells could withstand very little electricity, far less than normal healthy cells. So he set about mildly electrocuting his patients and even had some successes. Contreras feels that magnets could do a considerably better job!

The coming cancer cure
And so to his book that he is over here promoting *The Coming Cancer Cure*. In line with his beliefs he praises Gerson, decries the total lack of spending on cancer prevention, laments the declining nourishment values of modern diets and provides an overview of some future possible 'cures' for cancer.

Whilst the book's title is upbeat about finding a cancer 'cure', he himself is far more cynical and he tells the story of treating a congressman. When they discussed his hopes for an eventual cure, he was told that if he took a total cure to the USA President tomorrow, he'd "probably be killed!" "Cancer is such big business in the USA", he says, "bigger than Ford, General Motors and the rest. Imagine the job losses, the losses to the economy!".

Indeed in a number of our conversations he cites 'money' as the reason things do or do not happen.

Future perfect
Contreras has two more books planned; one a 40 year history of The Oasis of Hope, the other one on breast cancer. We

discuss the **icon** article, 'Oestrogen – the killer in our midst' and he tells me the treatment for breast cancer is simple: anti-oestrogen. We discuss prostate cancer about which he feels the same, however he adds the point that no one ever died of prostate cancer. He clearly feels that a lot of scare mongering exists.

Does he want a wave of new 'Oases' around the world? Yes, he'd love it. He has been trying to tie up a deal in England for 6 months but they haven't quite overcome funding issues. He has hopes for a hospital in Korea and maybe something in Japan. The Mexican wave is about to encompass the world.

Dr Francisco Contreras is a polite man. The word 'charm' springs into your mind after just a few minutes with him; then 'knowledge'; then 'passion'. It is important to remember he is Mexican, and the hospital started as a hospital for the Mexican poor. This is definitely not another case of Americans being driven over the border by vested interests.

It is clear that his open-minded approach to cancer results in truly integrated cancer treatments and we applaud him for that. Dr Francisco Contreras is undoubtedly one of **icon's** icons and we salute him on behalf of all our readers touched by cancer.

13 Metabolic therapy and the causes of cancers

Dr Paul Layman

icon September 2003

"What did your consultant say was the cause of your cancer?"

"He didn't say"

"Do you think he knows?

"I don't think so"

"Did he advise you on nutrition?"

"No"

"Did he suggest any supplements or stress management?"

"No"

"If he doesn't know what causes cancers, how come he's giving you all these powerful drugs, and burning radiation, with all the possible side effects?"

"When you put it that way, it doesn't sound very rational!"

The disclaimer – if this upsets you, then you may not want to read further. It upsets me as a doctor working outside the NHS. Maybe you might like to consider these things and put them in the mind's computer – if it "does not compute" then leave it.

Also all male gender pronouns can be considered to be female gender pronouns too, and most singulars as multiples. And not forgetting that none of this may be construed as medical advice and as always you can make your own investigations and do what you feel drawn to, rather than what a relative or even a medical professional tells you that "this is the only way".

Metabolic therapy
Moving away from these abstracts, 'Metabolic Therapy' was coined apparently by Dr Ernesto Contreras, the father of Dr Francisco Contreras at the Oasis of Hope Hospital in Mexico, many years ago. 'Metabolic' comes from metabolism, which describes the turnover of foods, hormones and all the molecules of the body. Catabolism is the breaking down of body tissues in illness, for example. Anabolism is the term for building up, as in anabolic steroids, which some ill-advised athletes have used to put on muscle bulk. They are also used in some farming practices to fatten up beef.

So, it is becoming recognised that cancer like most other illnesses is a metabolic disease. In other words one bacteria or one virus or one poison does not cause it. It is the result of a gradual deterioration of the body's metabolism until the immune system can no longer re-cycle the abnormal cells.

Secrets revealed
Here's a well-kept secret that could make the difference between life and death. We're all getting cancer cells all the time! Of the hundreds of thousands of cells created by our body every day some will be malformed, won't mature, won't die when they are supposed to, and will multiply without stopping. These are all the characteristics of cancer cells.

On a recent BBC Horizon programme, they showed brilliant graphics of how antioxidants prevented the damage of free radical 'hits'. These 'hits' are visualised as little bombs damaging our cells, particularly the young ones. The 'hits' come from radiation, poisons in the blood, and all sorts of other stresses, and are happening all the time, especially in our modern society. As the body becomes more damaged so the free radical activity becomes insufficient and the immune system suffers. Abnormal cells are not recycled and tumours develop.

Charlotte Gerson, daughter of the famous Dr Max Gerson and his Gerson Therapy, said that the Liver Function Tests do not show abnormality until at least 70 per cent of the liver is damaged. This can be shown with liver biopsies, and comparing organ damage with the blood tests. This raises the possibility that many of us are walking around sub-optimally healthy, in other words, only just managing to get out of bed in the morning, do a day's work and crash out in the evening, to repeat the spiral the next days and weeks, until we develop a specific illness.

Accumulating damage

So the next well-kept secret is that cancer like other diseases is a **build up** of damage to the immune system and the metabolic processes, from many causes. For each person it will be different, and some causes may be more obvious than others.

"I think my cancer may have developed after my husband died, because of the stress."

"Nonsense, stress has nothing to do with cancers – it's the genes."

The metabolic processes are not rocket science … Anything, including stress that damages the immune system is harmful to our cells. A build up of harmful effects leads to cancer and other diseases.

"Do you suggest any particular diet?"

"No, eat what you like, and my dietician recommends 'Wotsits' to put on weight (true story), and my oncology nurse advises to 'avoid fruit and vegetables, and eat white bread (true story), to avoid fibre that can aggravate radiation or chemotherapy induced diarrhoea."

"But the cancer help centres are recommending an organic vegan diet."

"Diet has nothing to do with cancers."

or

"I know that breast cancer is caused partly by the hormone effects of pesticides and weedkillers, but the patients are not ready to be told that!" (true story)

In a well planned Metabolic Therapy all the causes of the immune system deterioration are recognised and reversed as far as possible.

A rational programme
The first stage is often to take a range of nutritional supplements that have been missing from, or low in, our diets for decades. This is easy-peasy.

The second is to dramatically change the way we eat, moving away from fats and greasy chemicalised foods to fresh healthy organic produce. This is more of a challenge. There are so many preservatives in our food that undertakers are noticing that bodies are taking twice as long to decompose!

Reviewing the range of radiations we are subjecting ourselves to is a little more involved. The mobile phone issue will not go away, and we are living in 'electro-smog', from TV and radio waves, power lines, nuclear power station radiation – has everybody forgotten Chernobyl? The sheep farmers in Wales haven't forgotten their livelihood was contaminated. Reducing exposure is worth looking at from add-on devices for computers and phones, to considerations of geopathy (more later).

Radiation we know builds up, and that is why the X-ray technicians wear their dosage badges. If the dose accumulates beyond a critical level they need to move away from the X-ray machines. Sitting at a computer all day will allow a faster build up than if the computer is away from the workstation and only accessed when needed, or put into 'hibernation' mode.

Stresses of modern days
The most difficult area people generally find to deal with is emotion.

Husband: "I'm not stressed in any way."

Wife: "Yes, you are – you're always grumpy, you've been biting your nails ever since I met you, and you drink far too much!"

This is a common scenario, which is another good reason why the family or partner/friend can usefully be included in the consultation. 'Denial' is valid and is such a strong defence to protect ourselves against the hurts and fears of life. However in the long term it becomes counter productive and has to be exposed for what it is, if we wish to make progress.

Fortunately in these busy times, there are modern techniques that are relatively quick and painless. The days of psychoanalysis weekly for twenty years are over. Believe it or not there are thousands of well-qualified therapists of all sorts just waiting for us to give them a call to bring in their skills.

We use Emotional Freedom Technique and MCH (Multidimensional Cellular Healing), plus counselling and group interactions as standard, but there are many other treatments that can be very supportive and gently remove the stigmas of years. We suggest people go by other people's recommendations, and treat themselves to "treatments" that are relaxing and encouraging.

Hugging – the way of the future
It's rather unusual, but we find our patients and staff like hugs. It's said that four hugs a day are a basic need, and twelve a day are necessary for growth. We get used to washing our shirts more often – the left shoulder tends to get tear stained. Isn't it strange how we have developed into a nation of non-touchers? There is a craving for getting back to natural touch and communication. It takes a little courage, but there are a few helpful guidelines.

If you feel you want to hug someone, ask if they would like a hug. The shock for mother-in-law when she is suddenly grappled may be too much.

Looking someone gently and directly into the eyes is a way to ease the inevitable hug.

Giving a little gift of a flower or sweetie is a way to help others appreciate themselves and give us a hug.

If it all goes wrong and you bang heads or get caught up in jewellery, just have a good laugh – it's just as therapeutic.

B-17 and pancreatic enzymes
A crucial part of the recycling of abnormal cells has to do with the natural destructive function of cyanide. Fortunately nature built in protective mechanisms when designing the immune system. The B-17 molecule, variously called amygdalin (which is detailed in the doctor's pharmacopoeia) or laetrile, contains a carbon and nitrogen atom linked to form the cyanide radical. These cyanide radicals are very common in our foodstuffs from broccoli (isothiocyanates), to vitamin B-12 (cyanocobalamin), and as amygdalin in apple pips, pear pips, tapioca, millet, buckwheat and hundreds.

You can add hydrochloric acid, nitric acid or sulphuric acid to amygdalin and it won't release cyanide. The CN group is tightly protected with two sugar molecules and another complex that becomes benzaldehyde later. The only time this cyanide becomes active is when it comes into contact with cancer cells, which, because they are abnormally functioning have an enzyme B-glucosidase, and this breaks the molecule.

Pharmaceutical companies are well aware of this and have produced a synthetic drug called 'AGENT' (Antibody guided enzyme nitrile therapy) to have a very similar effect. As yet it has been only tested on mice, and exactly how much resemblance has a mouse to a man? They don't generally eat hamburgers and have mother-in-laws...

Pancreatic enzymes
Two of the biggest scourges of the Western world involve the pancreas. Sugar diabetes, as we know, is a disorder of the hormone function of the pancreas, largely due to the over consumption of refined sugars, but also linked to mineral deficiencies and long-term emotional issues.

Cancers also involve the pancreas, this time the digestive enzymes. Over the last century as the incidence of cancers has gone up from one in a hundred of the population to the epidemic of one in two that we have now, the meat consumption of the western world has exploded. Could these be linked perhaps? Remembering that all diseases are multi-factorial and involve a build up of many poisons, radiation and stresses, still animal products have a huge part to play in the damage to the pancreas.

The science suggests that enzymes such as Trypsin and Chymotrypsin have several actions. As well as digesting our steak and chips, café latte and fish fingers, part of them is absorbed into the bloodstream. Cancer cells seem to be protected by a protein coating, and eating through this protection allows access to the B-17, and hence the killing effect of cyanide. The addition of pancreatic enzymes, in between meals, appears to be effective in helping the Metabolic Therapy.

Minerals and vitamins

A huge number of nutritional companies have a bewildering variety of supplements on the market and all of them have a good line in persuasion – how does one choose? You can use a pin and blindfold, or use some common sense!

Minerals and microminerals needed in our diet number around 65, so buying the odd Selenium or Calcium doesn't make much sense. We should look at the way nature provides these items, and they're in small quantities and all jumbled up. In addition they are in **food**, so it is not so natural to eat ground up rocks or iron filings to get the minerals.

We feel that liquid colloidal minerals are a good and safe source of supplements, as are some of the 'superfoods' and 'food state' varieties. Each clinic and advisor will have their own preferences, based on their understanding and experience. It is not so important which variety we choose, as to get on and start supplementing – they don't do any good just sitting on the shelf. As time goes by, so we become more selective, but that's small print stuff – just get started!

Some of you will be tuned in enough to know what is doing your body good and what is passing through without any effect – that's the best way to be, but it takes practice and some are more skilled than others at this.

Coffee enemas

That's right, upside down coffee – without milk and sugar! Enemas are nothing new and have been done for thousands of years to cleanse the bowel.

Using organic coffee is a remarkable technique used extensively in the Gerson Therapy. The liver is stimulated to produce more bile outflow, carrying with it toxins and poisons. Telling people about this causes more laughs than any of our other techniques, so it must be good medicine.

Glyconutrients

There is an impressive body of scientific data about these 'super sugars'. They don't come in Mars Bars or cream cakes, but were components of our diets before we became fully processed, frozen, microwaved and TV dinnered.

Interestingly Aloe Vera has one of these glyconutrients as does Noni Juice. Glucosamine has been shown to be useful in arthritic conditions. Mannose and Fucose have some interesting effects on cancer cells, and these are natural items which look to us as having great potential.

Progesterone

This is a human hormone that balances and counteracts the effects of oestrogens. Dr John Lee has done amazing work in revealing its secrets to the world, but it is still a mystery to most medical professionals. There is a good scientific database about Progesterone, but also much confusion about this natural hormone and its unnatural synthetic relatives that are found in HRT (Hormone Replacement Therapy).

Both the Glyconutrients and Progesterone, as well as other anti-cancer agents, have the ability to regulate cell growth, to persuade cells to die at their allotted time, and also to encourage naughty adolescent cells to mature into fully functioning members of society! And scientists are aware of the genes P53 and BCl2 that have particular influence on these processes.

As you can see, there is an amazing amount that can be done to help yourself or your loved ones, at whatever stage. Also remember, like in the song, 'There is a season, turn, turn, turn, and a time for every purpose under heaven.' There is a time for striving and a time for letting go, and we're all here to help each other to that end.

Quick – hug someone before the feeling wears off!

14 C for yourself (vitamin C)

Chris Woollams

icon January 2004

Vitamin C, ascorbic acid, is so important to your health that a human will die within a few months if it is not included in the diet. Humans, chimpanzees, fruit bats and guinea pigs are the only mammals that cannot synthesise it. If sufficient of the vitamin is not included in the diet, the feet, hands and gums swell, and then this spreads to the rest of the body. In 1589 these symptoms were defined as 'scurvy' and by 1593 Sir Richard Hawkins, desperate because he'd lost 10,000 men to the disease noted that oranges and lemons reversed the disease. His cure, though, fell out of favour (costing many more lives) until revived in the mid-1700s when a surgeon Dr Lind realised that if men ate two oranges and one lemon a day, within a week they had fully recovered. In 1804 the British Navy ordered lime juice for all its sailors and the nickname 'limeys' was born.

By 1911 it was fully recognised that scurvy was a vitamin deficiency although it was not until 1928 that it was first isolated as vitamin C by the Nobel Prize winner Dr Szent-Györgyi.

Recommended Daily Allowance
The League of the United Nations recommended that everybody should take 30 mgs per day, as this was the threshold level to prevent scurvy. By 1974 The National Research Council amended this slightly to Infants: 35mgs, Children: 40mgs, Adults: 45mgs.

However as we will see this is woefully inadequate for sustained good health and in the cancer prevention process.

What does vitamin C actually do?
Vitamin C plays a number of quite varied but fundamental roles in the body.

1 Ascorbic acid is required for the synthesis of collagen and connective tissue
Collagen strengthens tendons, cartilage, bones, arteries and veins, for example.

In 1933 Ewan Cameron, a surgeon at the Vale of Leven Hospital Scotland, presented a theory about how vitamin C might act to prevent tumour development in a paper 'Hyaluronidase and Cancer'.

All malignant tumours probably produce two enzymes, hyaluroldase and collagenase, which weaken the connective tissues and the 'glue' between cells around the tumour, thus allowing the rogue cells to spread. The theory ran that vitamin C was an inhibitor of these enzymes and a possible treatment to restrict tumours and stop their growth might be vitamin C **megadoses** of 10gms and above (see later).

2 Ascorbic acid strengthens the immune system
Early studies showed that vitamin C increased the body's resistance to a cold; in stressful situations like surgery, burns or wounds the levels of vitamin C in the blood fall; and in 1943 Cottingham and Mills show that phagocytosis actually uses vitamin C to ingest and eradicate bacteria.

Indeed in 1990 Hernanz et al showed that vitamin C was important for antiviral and phagocytic activity. By 1996 Jariwalla and Harakeh had shown its immunostimulant effect on lymphocytes.

De la Frente, Ferrandex Burgos and Solex showed that a combination of 1gm of vitamin C and 200mgs of vitamin E improved lymphocytes, neutrophils and phagocytes. Another study by Jariwalla showed that vitamin C boosts phagocytosis and T-lymphocytes (the immune cells that recognise and hunt down rogue invading cells). Lympocytes are now known to store large amounts of vitamin C ready to attack forming cancer cells (Riordan, Aidan Clinic, Arizona).

The most crucial study was probably the 1973 study by Hume and Weyers that showed 250mgs was not enough to support the phagocytes activity and that 1gm was suggested, rising to 6gms at the first sign of a cold.

Finally vitamin C is known to stimulate the production of interferon which helps protect cells against viral and cancer attack.

3 Ascorbic acid is a powerful antioxidant
A number of studies (Ginter 1970, 1973, 1975; Spittle 1971) have shown that vitamin C can counteract saturated fats being converted by oxidation into dangerous peroxides. Meydani et al (1995) and Pike and Chandra (1995) both showed that antioxidant diets centering on vitamin C produced less illness overall.

Ascorbic acid is a weak acid, a little stronger than vinegar (acetic acid) and is a reducing agent – it donates electrons and hydrogen atoms. It seems to protect cells from oxidative damage, and it interferes with the production and activity of free radicals.

4 Ascorbic acid can inactivate bacteria and viruses
The action against free radicals seems to parallel ascorbic acid's action against bacteria and viruses. Phagocytosis seems to actually use ascorbate to deactivate bacteria.

Akira Murata showed that ascorbate could inactivate many of the viruses that attack bacteria. Intravenous injections of 20gms of sodium ascorbate inactivated many types of virus within 20 minutes. Murata, Kitagawa and Suromo (1971) showed that ascorbate needs free oxygen present. Ascorbate reduces the oxygen to a free radical, which destroys the nucleic acid of the virus (Pauling 1976).

Dr Morishige of Fukuoka, Japan used 10gms of ascorbate to treat measles, mumps, herpes and viral meningitis (Murata 1975). As far back as 1937, Boissevain and Spillane had showed vitamin C inhibits the growth of Tuberculosis bacteria.

5   Vitamin C reduces stomach cancer risk
This is a very specific benefit. Vitamin C helps block the formation of nitrosamines, potential carcinogens formed in the stomach from nitrates in food and produced by microbes.

6   Vitamin C minimises allergic reactions
It interferes with the production of histamines, released by the immune system in response to an allergen, thus reducing allergic reaction.

How much should you take?
Linus Pauling, two–time Nobel Prize winner, first developed an interest in vitamin C in the 1960s after meeting Irwin Stone, a biochemist who had been studying the vitamin since the 1930s.

Stone had a view that since humans were one of only four groups of mammals unable to synthesise vitamin C for themselves, this 'problem' had risen through genetic deficiency and it was up to us to correct it ourselves!

Using studies on rats and extrapolating the results Stone concluded that humans needed 1.4 to 4.0gms per day (Hager).

Pauling took this work forward with a number of people. He noted that animals that do make their own make it constantly out of dextrose in the liver or kidney. Vitamin C is water-soluble and can wash out of general tissues in just 3 hours. It is not stored and cells need a constant supply.

Aspirin and the antibiotic tetracycline increase the rate of destruction of vitamin C in the body. Oestrogen, especially from HRT or the pill, increases excretion in the urine. People with diabetes, people who are stressed, smokers and people who drink lots of alcohol all have lower vitamin C levels.

But the real problem is the recommended level required. The RDA has been set at the level required simply to avoid scurvy. There is a plethora of evidence that this is way too low to avoid other everyday diseases. Worse, when Pauling studied the subject back in 1976 he concluded one third of those studied were not even getting the RDA of 45mgs!

Pauling in 1976 said that the desired daily level was somewhere between 250mgs and 10gms. There are claims that too much can cause liver damage, and even one that it causes cancer. Neither has been substantiated.

Vitamin C and cancer
Neil Riordan at the Aidan Clinic, Arizona has noted that 46 per cent of breast cancer sufferers are vitamin C deficient, some even to the point of scurvy (*British Journal of Cancer* Vol 84, 11).

There are a great number of studies which show that cancer sufferers have lowered vitamin C levels in their blood. That it lowers cancer risk for breast, cervix, colon, rectum, mouth, lung, prostate, stomach and oesophagus is very well documented (e.g. Levin, *National Academy of Sciences*) Vol 93, 8 1996; *Block Nutrition Review* Vol 50, 7 1992; Frei, *Journal of the American Medical Association*) Vol 97, 1994; Uddin, *Comprehensive Therapy* Vol 2.1, 1995).

The controversy centres on whether or not large or 'megadoses' can actually cure cancer:

In 1974 Cameron and Campbell took 50 terminal cancer patients and gave them 10gms intravenously of sodium ascorbate. All had been given less than 3 months to live, a half survived 361 days on average with 5 people surviving an average of 610 days.

They requested that the National Cancer Institute conduct proper clinical trials – a double blind study. For some reason or other this was denied. So Pauling and Cameron repeated the experiment with 100 terminal cancer patients comparing them with control groups of 1000 people in all. Whilst the entire 1000 control group died, 18 of the group receiving vitamin C survived, and 5 of these appeared to overcome the disease.

In 1978 Pauling and Cameron repeated this in a second study, this time taking 9 control groups each with similar cancers to the test group. As in the previous tests, the patients taking vitamin C had renewed vigour and energy and their quality of life improved. Whilst the entire control group died, the vitamin C group lived 300 days on average and 5 patients survived for 16 months.

Morishiga and Murata did a similar study in Japan with 99 terminal cancer patients and concluded that 10gm 'megadose' intravenous vitamin C gave a threefold uplift in survival rate.

One caveat to all this is that vitamin C megadoses do not seem to work anything like as well if the patient has had chemotherapy. In Cameron's experiments only 4 people had had chemotherapy. But in 1978 the Mayo Clinic conducted double blind tests on vitamin C (Cregan et al) using 60 subjects of which 52 had had chemotherapy. They concluded that their results could not endorse the Scottish findings; and observers pointed the finger at chemotherapy, which was felt to impede the vitamin C effect.

However, Cameron's hyaluronidase theory seems to be sound. For example, the speed of breast cancer spread is believed to be about free-radical damage and is drastically reduced by vitamin C (Malins, *National Academy of Sciences* Vol 93, March 1996).

Dr Hoffer of Victoria, Canada took Pauling and Cameron's beta-carotene minerals. He showed there was a 16 times greater survival rate in the test group over the control group!

In 1993 Pauling and Cameron gave 3gms of vitamin C to people who had pre-malignant polyps in their intestines. In this study half the patients had their polyps disappear.

One point worth stressing is that vitamin C taken orally is normally used when the doses are small. 'Megadose vitamin C' involves intravenous injection of ascorbate. Paydayatly and Levine conducted research in 2001 showing there was no benefit in high oral doses. There is some evidence (confirmed by the Dove Clinic) that megadose vitamin C (75 gms level) should not be used on patients with primary or secondary brain tumours as it causes astrocytosis – i.e. the spreading of the tumour.

Riordan took the view that vitamin C brings about cancer cell death because large doses build up hydrogen peroxide in cancer cells. Normal cells contain catalase, an enzyme that breaks this down protecting the cells. If you are taking high levels of vitamin C you should increase magnesium levels to avoid kidney stones.

Antioxidants and chemo or radiotherapy?
Which brings us to the issue of should you supplement if you are having chemo or radiotherapy. Riordan's research, above, seems to say clearly that with vitamin C you should.

In 1999 Gotlieb went further; with Kedar Prasad, Professor of Radiology at the University of Colorado, Denver, they showed that high dose vitamin C, as well as other antioxidants, can protect healthy cells which regulate their uptake levels during treatment. Whereas, Prasad is quite clear, cancer cells cannot regulate uptake and this aids their death. Whilst he is actually against high doses of vitamin C because of possible toxicity in the liver, he believes C, E and beta-carotene are highly protective. (Smokers might be wary of beta-carotene.)

Foods for vitamin C (mgs)

raw pommelo	370
blackcurrants, 1 cup	200
guava, half cup	150
red pepper, half cup	140
fresh orange juice (8 fluid ozs)	120
brussel sprouts, cooked, 1 cup	100
papaya, 1 cup	90
strawberries, 1 cup	75
brussel sprouts, raw, 1 cup	75
pineapple	70
kiwi	70
grapefruit (8 oz)	70
green snap peas	50
tomato juice (8 oz)	40
raw broccoli	40

In Boik's book 'Natural Compounds in Cancer Therapy' he reviews both *in vitro* and *in viro* studies that antioxidants actually **improve** the success of chemotherapy and radiotherapy contrary to popular mythology.

Cooking reduces vitamin C content by half. Vitamin C is also destroyed by poor storage. A potato will lose 70 per cent of its vitamin C over the first 5 days after being dug up.

Anything else?

Well now you come to mention it, vitamin C has been shown to neutralise the action of aflatoxin B, the toxin of parasites in your body. This might explain some of the benefit of vitamin C in terminal cancer cases. After all, the World Health Organisation believes at least 15–20 per cent of all cancers are caused by infection.

And finally, vitamin C is highly influential as part of an anti-aging programme. The National Institute of Aging showed that people who took vitamin C and E supplements had a 50 per cent lower risk of dying prematurely. This was backed up by a Californian study, which showed that a supplement of 750mgs a day reduced the risk of dying prematurely by 60 per cent. A third US study showed that 1 gm of vitamin C and 1000 IUs of vitamin C was preventative for Alzheimer's.

Environmental pollutants can cause the breakdown of vitamin C in the body.

If you're still with us after all this, it looks like a 1gm Ester-C supplement per day might be no bad thing, but taken as four lots of 250 mgs across the day.

15 Are there safer ways of killing cancer cells than chemotherapy?
Vitamin C megadoses

Dr Julian Kenyon

icon February 2003

Conventional oncology largely uses chemotherapy to destroy cancer cells. There can be no doubt that chemotherapy works, and that in any cancer case, cancer cells need destroying. Chemotherapy is backed by high quality clinical trials and has been studied extensively for nearly 40 years. Practically every known solid tumour has a solid evidence-base and the oncologist will be able to give you a pretty accurate percentage success rate of any particular treatment regime, in any particular solid cancer. However, clearly, chemotherapy has a downside as it's a highly toxic treatment and in many patients is poorly tolerated, and there are studies in the conventional oncology literature that imply that a significant number of patients can die of chemotherapy, as opposed to the cancer. A recent play televised at peak viewing time on BBC2 in December 2002, called 'WIT', portrayed a harrowing drama about a woman, an English Professor, dying of cancer. The heroine was brilliantly acted by Emma Thompson. The dramatic high point of the drama was when the heroine said to camera. "It's not the cancer that's killing me, it's the treatment".

"Everyone in medicine understands that a great deal of uncertainty about what to do for people, will always remain in any illness. Human disease and lives are too complicated for reality to be otherwise". This is taken from a recent book by Atul Gawande entitled *Complications: A Surgeon's Notes on an*

Imperfect Science. Cancer is just such a complex illness. Current medicine is evidence based as outlined in the first part of this article on chemotherapy. However, what happens if you do not wish to partake of the conventional treatment option such as chemotherapy? Are there alternatives? Yes, there are, but they currently have a poor evidence base, and are never likely to have the quality of the evidence base that backs chemotherapy. Providing the cancer sufferer knows what the evidence is, then they can make treatment choices on an informed consent basis. In my view it's unethical for patients to be offered any of these treatments without as good an evidence-base as chemotherapy, other than on an informed consent basis. High dose intravenous vitamin C is one of these treatments, and we use it extensively in our clinic. It is one of our most effective treatments. Clearly because of the poor evidence base we largely see chemotherapy and radiotherapy failures, but interestingly enough those patients who deliberately seek us out and wish to try these approaches as a first line option, tend to be the 'more well-informed' public, and amongst these, number some doctors, which is indeed a curious situation.

Vitamin C (ascorbic acid) is a major water-soluble antioxidant with a variety of biological functions. It may be important in maintaining proper immune cell function. Even though vitamin C commonly functions as an antioxidant is can also act as a pro-oxidant, that is actually oxidising tissues, which is what chemotherapy does. Vitamin C converts free radicals into hydrogen peroxide, a molecule that can damage cell membranes if not neutralised by an enzyme inside the cell called catalase. Tumour cells have 10–100 times less catalase than normal cells, and are therefore more sensitive than normal to hydrogen peroxide. Vitamin C accumulates in solid tumours at concentrations higher than those in surrounding normal tissue. The accumulation of vitamin C preferentially in cancer tissues has raised concerns that vitamin C may provide tumours with antioxidant protection from chemotherapeutic agents. In practice therefore, the avoidance of vitamin C and indeed all antioxidants, when going through a chemotherapy programme, is important.

To obtain vitamin C levels at pro-oxidant levels, at which level it destroys cancer cells, is only achievable by intravenous infusion. Plasma levels of vitamin C between 300–400 milligrams per 100cc are what is required in order to kill significant numbers of cancer cells. This requires intravenous infusions of 75 grams of vitamin C (in some cases less, depending on the size of the patient and the tumour cell mass), infused intravenously on a daily basis for three weeks in order to be able to attain these plasma levels. It's important to realise that the highest plasma level of vitamin C achievable in humans using oral supplementation is 4.5 milligrams per 100cc. Many studies have been done on this approach in the laboratory and Phase I and Phase II clinical trials have been completed on this approach. (Phase II clinical trials have been carried out in Nebraska, USA and are about to be published.) Phase III clinical studies are in discussion.

Our most common protocol is the use of 75 grams of vitamin C in sterile water, with a number of minerals, particularly magnesium, zinc, chromium, selenium, B-12 and some B vitamins. The patient is infused over 2? hours daily for 3 weeks (excluding weekends). The vitamin C level at the end of the infusion course is tested and if this is sufficiently high then some significant tumour kill has happened. If it isn't, then this regime may have to be repeated. The advantage of using this approach is that it doesn't carry the downsides of chemotherapy, and can be repeated many times. The main downside is that if we are working with patients who have fluid accumulation in the chest, say from a lung cancer, or fluid accumulation in the abdomen say from ovarian cancer, then the fluid load that these intravenous infusions involve can make these situations worse. So in those patients we choose other safe options to kill cancer cells.

Concurrently with the high dose intravenous vitamin C, we use supplements, the most important of which is lipoic acid. Lipoic acid has been found to enhance the cancer killing effect of vitamin C, and the mechanism for this is unknown.

The only side effect we see in this treatment is tiredness due to tumour cell death, as well as increased fluid accumulation in particular groups of patients, as mentioned above.

So in conclusion, even though chemotherapy has such a high quality evidence-base, it doesn't mean that other, less well-researched treatments do not also work.

16 A review of key vitamins and minerals. But do they work on cancer?

Drawn from articles in **icon**
by Chris Woollams

(a) Vitamin A
icon September 2003

When it comes to cancer, it's confusing
The overwhelming conclusion when studying vitamin A (as opposed to Beta-carotene) is that where cancer is concerned the jury is out. There are research papers that conclude it is helpful; and there are papers that conclude it has no effect. Vitamin A does, however, have clear health giving properties. It helps strengthen the immune system (especially the white cells) and, in particular, it strengthens epithelial tissues (and, by implication, blocking the process by which many cancers form). Vitamin A also helps the action of vitamin C.

The history
Egyptian documents dating from 1500 BC tell that squeezing the juice of a fried or roasted animal liver directly into the eyes could cure people suffering night blindness. Hippocrates refined this a little and simply suggested eating liver to treat the condition. By the twelfth century healers had identified that foods like fish and egg yolks aided human growth and healing. By 2001 some researchers in America were linking high blood serum vitamin A levels to protection against both breast and prostate cancers.

The vitamin

Vitamin A itself is actually a family of fat-soluble vitamins, including retinol and retinoic acid. They are often dubbed 'pre-formed vitamin A'.

Vitamin A helps the normal development and growth of bones, it is essential for all cell differentiation, epithelial tissues, visual function and reproductive function. It is also noted as an anti-ageing agent. It is not an antioxidant.

Pure vitamin A is usually only available on prescription as it is toxic in regular, but not large amounts. The only sources of pre-formed vitamin A are 'animal', for example, fish oils, especially cod liver oil, whole milk and liver. Many fortified foods, for example breakfast cereals, contain it.

It is stored in the liver, from where it is released in times of shortage. Large doses of vitamin A cause liver toxicity – the symptoms include a yellowing of skin or eyes, rashes, fatigue, headaches and blurred vision.

Vitamin A is lost during food preparation, cooking and storage.

USA RDA for vitamin A is 1000 retinol equivalents, where 1 RE equals 3.33 International Units, i.e. 3,333 IUs per day. An absolute maximum of 100,000 IUs is set for vitamin A daily consumption.

The beta-carotene confusion

A second way of increasing levels of vitamin A in the body is via its precursors, the carotenes – also called provitamin A. This allows your body to convert the precursors into vitamin A, as and when needed. However polyunsaturated fats block the conversion unless there are good supplies of other antioxidants present. In other words, the best way to keep your vitamin A level up is to take it in beta-carotene, with other antioxidants.

Does it help in cancer?
There are many reports of beta-carotene as an antioxidant helping in cancer prevention and treatment. Unfortunately some of these confuse the issue with vitamin A.

"Unlike beta-carotene vitamin A is not an antioxidant, so its benefits relate to its possible roles in reversing tumour development and boosting immune function" (McDonald).

"The association of vitamin A and cancer was initially reported in 1926 when rats, fed a vitamin A deficient diet, developed gastric carcinomas" (Loescher, *Vitamin Therapy for Advanced Cancer*).

The first investigation showing a relationship between vitamin A and human cancer was performed in 1941 by Abelsetal who found low plasma vitamin A levels in patients with gastro-intestinal cancers.

T E Moon and colleagues (South West Stem Cancer Prevention Study Group, *Cancer Epidemiological Biomarkers* Prev 1997) conducted a randomised double blind, controlled trial on retinol supplementation with melanomas. This study concluded that supplementation with 25,000 IUs of retinol per day was effective in preventing squamous cell carcinoma.

Finally McDonald concluded "vitamin A has the potential to reverse pre-cancerous lesions".

Or maybe not?
Olson has observed that, for example, some studies show a connection between serum retinol levels and prostate cancer whilst others do not. He acknowledges that vitamin A is essential for cell differentiation (an important step in the cancer process) but that there is no *consistent* association established with the cancer role.

There are as many studies with no result concluded, as there are suggestions of an effect.

The last word?
It is possible that the type of vitamin A is the crucial factor.

Proponents of vitamin A's success argue that on top of cell differentiation promotion, vitamin A also inhibits cellular proliferation (Baumann did research on breast cancer cells).

Spencer argued that there are decreases in similar metastases if retinoids were used alongside other treatments after the primary tumour was removed.

Now new research studies announced in February 2003 by Dr Wann Ki Hong at the University of Texas believe retinoic acid is the active ingredient, and they have formulated a drug from it that seems to be effective.

The study involved former smokers. Smoking causes genetic damage, which takes time to disappear, leaving the ex-smoker at risk. It is known that retinoic acid is essential for the epithelial cells in the lungs to function normally by activating retinoic acid receptors. Loss of the receptors leads to lung cancer. Dr Wann Ki Hong and his team have developed a drug derivative of retinoic acid, which showed a 7 per cent risk reduction.

Dr Julia Sharp of Cancer Research UK said, on hearing about the trial, that vitamin A derivatives might have the potential to help repair cells damaged by smoking.

So vitamin A might not work after all, but a drug based on it might.

You'll have to draw your own conclusions on this one!

Vitamin A and Beta-carotene
icon September 2003

An alternative view
Right now, in the USA, a lady called Mary L Cupp is helping her State Representative draft a bill about the obligation of doctors to their patients. Her story concerns vitamin A.

Mary's story began in 1986 when she sought dietary advice from a holistic, but fully qualified US doctor who recommended a strict vegetarian, dairy-free diet.

Over the two years that followed, Mary's health deteriorated markedly until she developed anaemia, gastrointestinal bloating and other problems. A chiropractor recommended iron tablets. A short while later Mary developed a severe uterine haemorrhage. Going back to the original doctor, the recommendation was a hysterectomy but Mary refused. She was given medication and the recommendation was repeated several times over the four years that followed. One day Mary was admitted to hospital with life-threatening bleeding. She had the operation.

Several months after the hysterectomy, Mary discovered an article about a 1977 South African medical journal study of vitamin A as therapy for excessive bleeding. The study resulted in a 92.5 per cent cure rate. The article further covered the use of vitamin A at Johannesburg General Hospital with a documented 92 per cent cure rate over a 10-year period. (Excessive bleeding is the main symptom that leads to hysterectomies.)

Mary did more research and discovered that the extreme vegetarian diet recommended by her doctor could deplete vitamin A, which can only be found in animal products. Worse, people with low thyroid function are unable to convert beta-carotene into vitamin A. Coincidentally patients with low thyroid function often have excess bleeding and a higher risk of reproductive organ surgery. Soy foods, which Mary used to replace dairy, can depress thyroid function. Furthermore vitamin A aids the absorption of iron and the building of blood.

Mary started to take vitamin A supplements and her health improved. She learned that vitamin A is definitely connected to the health of the gastrointestinal tract, and she followed the work of Dr Weston Price, whose work emphasises the need for both vitamins A and D in the diet. Her corrective vitamin A intake was 100,000 IUs.

(b) Beta-carotene
icon August 2003

Carotenoids are good for you
Beta-carotene is a member of the Carotenoids family. In all there are over 500 members including, lutein, cryptoxanthia, alpha-carotene, zeaxanthin and lycopene.

As a rule of thumb, carotenoids are found in dark green leaves and in bright orange, yellow and red vegetables. Rather unsurprisingly, the name derives from the fact that they were first discovered in carrots.

Leaving aside lycopene, which we will deal with in a future article and is found in tomatoes, tomatoes, tomatoes and a little in pink grapefruit, carotenoids are most commonly found in bright coloured peppers, apricots, carrots, greens, kale, spinach, broccoli, sweet potato, fennel and pumpkins. Consuming an excess of beta-carotene either in supplement or natural form, has been know to impart a yellowish tint to the skin!

Beta-carotene seems to have three actions:

- It is an immune system booster
- It can act as antioxidant.
- It can convert in the body to vitamin A, a proven anti-cancer agent.

Beta-carotene the antioxidant
Every day the power stations in the cells produce waste by-products. Some of these are known as free radicals. The level of free radicals in the human body is worsened by 'bad' fat consumption, alcohol consumption and smoking. However excess exercise can also increase free radical levels.

A normal molecule has paired electrons, a free radical has a lone singleton looking to rip an electron off any molecule it passes; a cell membrane, an immune cell, even your DNA. Antioxidants neutralize free radicals preventing them doing harm. Beta-carotene is fat-soluble and like vitamin E protects cellular membranes.

Beta-carotene and the immune system
Many laboratories have linked free radicals to the anti-ageing decline in the immune system. Dr Simin Meydani at Tufts studied the effects of 50 mg daily supplementation, showing that this produced much higher levels of natural killer cells than in normal adults.

Beta-carotene and vitamin A
As we said, there are a number of reports on the anti-cancer benefits of vitamin A. However vitamin A is toxic to the liver in large doses and it is often thought better to increase levels of beta-carotene and let the body convert the required levels. Beta-carotene itself is non-toxic. Now, whether the vitamin A or the beta-carotene is the strong anti-cancer agent is open to question . . .

Beta-carotene and cancer prevention
Care has to be taken when attributing anti-cancer benefits to beta-carotene, as it is the precursor of vitamin A, which has been known to inhibit cancers since the 1940s. Nevertheless there are over 200 studies showing positive benefit for beta-carotene in the fight against cancer.

A study that started in the 1970s in Switzerland and lasted 12 years concluded that men with a lower blood level of carotenoids had a higher cancer mortality rate. This was particularly true for cancer where the difference was 60 per cent. Beta-carotene is known to have a particularly strong protective effect on epithelial tissues e.g. the throat, intestines, lungs, colon and bladder.

In 1989 the University of Washington and the Fred Hutchinson

Cancer Research Centre linked high beta-carotene intake with lowered cervical cancer rates.

In Britain, 5004 women had samples of blood frozen and over a number of years their health was monitored by St Bartholomew's Hospital, London. Beta-carotene levels were almost 50 per cent higher in women without cancer than in the ones who developed breast cancer.

Another study showed that 44 per cent of people with colon cancer who were given 30 mg daily supplements had cancer inhibition after just two weeks. While researchers in Arizona showed supplementation, also using 30 mgs per day for pre-cancerous mouth lesions (leukoplakia), caused total or partial regression in 71 per cent of tumours.

After clinical trials on prostate, cervical, colon, melanoma and breast cancers, the US Prostate Cancer Research Institute concluded there was "sufficient reason to supplement with beta-carotene".

The downside?
Firstly there is some evidence that it can cause some liver toxicity in people whose alcohol consumption is high.

Then there are a couple of negative reports, where the sample studied were serious smokers, or exposed to asbestos.

A Finnish study, reported in the *Journal of the American Medical Association*, followed male smokers over 5–8 years. Those taking beta-carotene supplements had an 18 per cent higher lung cancer rate.

Another study, CARET, taking 18,000 women and men who smoked heavily or were exposed to asbestos showed an increased lung cancer rate of 28 per cent in the group that supplemented with beta-carotene/vitamin A.

In another study by Harvard University across 25 years and following 22,000 male physicians of ages between 40 and 84, those taking a supplement of 50 mgs per day gained neither benefit nor harm.

A conclusion drawn from this was that maybe the combined effect of a number of carotenoids was far more potent than taking a single supplement.

Another comment was that most beta-carotenes in supplements are synthetic and feature only one molecule (all trans beta-carotene) whereas the natural state incorporates two molecules (all trans and 9-cis beta-carotene).

It is highly likely that beta-carotene as a supplement may work best in combination with other antioxidants. As clearly mentioned it features in membranes with vitamin E. Indeed a five-year American study of 38,000 Chinese, reported in 1993, where beta-carotene, vitamin E and selenium were taken together resulted in a cancer mortality decrease of 13 per cent.

Supplementation
Beta-carotene is easily lost from the body and it should be taken as 3–5 mgs up to four times per day. Sometimes the packaging reports the dosage as International Units (IUs). 15 mgs is approximately 25,000 IUs.

(c) Vitamin B-12
icon May/June 2004

Why is it so important?
In recent years scientists have become more and more concerned about this vitamin and people over the age of 50 or people on strict vegetarian diets.

The vitamin is crucial to life and to general health, being involved in almost every cellular system in the body. The liver can store large amounts of B-12 so the occasional daily shortfall will not cause problems but increasingly, as more is known about the vitamin, deficiency concerns abound.

Vitamin B-12 or cobalamin, is water soluble and effective in very small doses. The recommended adult dose was in the region of just 3–5 micrograms per day until recently. However research with heart disease has shown levels of 100-400 micrograms are more in order. Heart attacks have been linked to low levels of vitamin B-12. (*American Journal of Epidemiology* Vol 143). The liver has such a large store of B-12 that deficiency symptoms might actually take 5 years to appear; however these are likely to include pernicious anaemia and brain damage.

The vitamin is known to help form and regenerate red blood cells. It helps prevent cardiovascular disease by lowering blood levels of homocysteine, it promotes growth and appetite in children, improves brainpower, concentration and memory, and is involved in a healthy nervous system. It also helps maintain a fatty tissue known as the myelin sheath surrounding nerve cells.

B-12 is also involved in the metabolism of carbohydrates and fats, but it is its importance in the synthesis of protein, DNA and RNA and its complex interconnection with folic acid, another B vitamin essential for accurate DNA replication that sparks a concern about its role in cancer. The body cannot use folic acid without B-12.

A little history
In the 1800s pernicious anaemia was widespread in Europe. A sore tongue and diarrhoea followed by nerve damage, mental disorder then death in the severest cases.

By the 1930s two Nobel Prize winners, William Murphy and George Minot, had clues to the disease noting that people who ate liver soon recovered. Vitamin B-12 was finally isolated after the war.

Sources
The best sources are all animal in origin, especially offal. Liver, kidneys, beef, poultry, milk, cheese, fish, egg yolks. Very little is lost in cooking, although microwaves have been shown to destroy 40 per cent of the B-12 content of foods.

Its enemies are acids and alkalis, oestrogen and alcohol. As it is water-soluble it can be flushed from the body. There have been no reported cases of toxicity from consumption of excess.

So has it actually been linked with cancer?
At least one research study (for example, Choi, Sang-Woo, *Nutrition Review* 57) has noted that women with breast cancer have lowered B-12 levels.

Whilst we may consume copious amounts of B-12 foods, extracting the vitamin from our ingested food can be a problem.

B-12 is a very large molecule. Firstly the stomach must secrete adequate amounts of acid plus the digestive enzyme pepsin. This may be a problem for older people and 20-30 per cent do not produce enough acid. 11 per cent of older people have B-12 deficiency (*Journal of American Geriatric Society* Vol 44). Whilst early symptoms are fatigue, memory loss and mental confusion, vitamin B-12 deficiency is linked to Alzheimer's and dementia (*Age and Ageing* Vol 23 pg 334). It will also be a problem where people mix carbohydrates and proteins in their mouth as carbohydrate arriving in the stomach demands a more alkaline environment, thus causing the stomach to receive conflicting messages. Separate your carbohydrate and protein meals.

Then this large molecule needs to combine with an 'intrinsic factor'; a protein, in order to be absorbed. However sometimes due to genetic defects, sometimes due to stomach injury, or even due to problems with the stomach lining, the 'intrinsic factor' effect is weak.

Researchers at the Turkish Military Academy identified that 77 per cent of people with vitamin B-12 deficiency had Helicobacter pylori. It is estimated that approximately 50 per cent of people in the West have the infection. In 1994 the International Agency for Research on Cancer declared Helicobacter pylori a Grade 1 (definite) carcinogen.

There is compelling evidence that *Helicobacter pylori* is linked to stomach and gastric cancers (e.g. Wang et al, *World of Gastroenterology* 2002: Dec 8) and to Lymphoma (e.g. Savia et al, Blood 1997; Feb). It is important to treat the original infection.

Helicobacter pylori is a spiral shaped bacterium that lives in the stomach and duodenum. Half a gallon of gastric juice is produced every day, but helicobacter pylori hides in the mucous membrane lining the stomach and surrounds itself with a neutralising fluid to prevent the gastric juice acid attack. Worse, the immune system sends white cells to kick out the invader but they cannot get through the stomach lining. So they collect and the immune response multiplies. Some bacterium die, helicobacter feeds on the nutrients, more white cells are sent and the vicious circle results in a peptic ulcer. Or worse.

Breath tests, endoscopy or Vega Testing can all establish its presence. Of course, orthodox medicine recommends a mixture of antibiotics to eradicate the bacterium. However, part of the orthodox cure seems to be acid lowering drugs, but this route would of course further reduce the B-12 ingestion. See a homeopath for a more rounded 'cure'. Lactobacillus suppresses Helicobacter, but does not eradicate it.

Essential B-12
73 per cent of vegetarians have been found to be deficient in B-12, even though the message about their non-B-12 diet is frequently repeated. Older people need more B-12. And it helps pregnant women, as B-12 is important in cell growth. Readers should refer to the section on Chlorella.

(d) Vitamin D
The vitamin that works like a hormone
icon February 2004

In 1919 Sir Edward Mellanby was working indoors with dogs and concluded that if they didn't get sunlight they developed bone disorders (typically 'rickets' in children). He further concluded that the essential action of fats preventing these problems was due to a vitamin; and that cod liver oil was a strong preventative agent. (More information on the importance of fish oils and omega 3 is contained in The Tree of Life: The Anti-Cancer Diet).

The chemical structure of this vitamin was identified in the 1930s by Professor A Windaus of the University of Göttingen, Germany. Thus vitamin D came about.

As we shall see, it is now known that this substance is not technically a vitamin at all, but acts as a classic steroid hormone! A detailed study of the biochemistry was not possible until the 1960s when 'radioactive vitamin D' could be prepared. Over the last few years researchers have come to learn completely new things about vitamin D, not least that the RDAs originally set for the prevention of rickets are woefully inadequate. Sadly they are still in place today.

What is it?
Vitamin D is an umbrella term for a number of fat-soluble chemicals called calciferols. Two are important to humans: D_2 is produced when ergosterol in plants is energised by the sun; D_3 or cholocalciferol is synthesied by the action of sunlight on our subcutaneous cholesterol layers.

The activity of vitamin D involves a five-step process: the generation or ingestion of D_3; liver metabolism to a hydroxyl form; circulation in blood; conversion to a double hydroxyl form in the kidneys; transport to nuclear receptor sites.

All this is a long way beyond those first views of vitamin D, where deficiencies were associated with rickets in the young and osteomalacia in adults.

Vitamin D and bones
Vitamin D is essential for maintaining bone density and preventing osteoporosis as it helps the absorption of bone-building materials calcium and phosphorus. In this action it is helped by magnesium. All these minerals are best absorbed from plant sources. Of course dairy foods also provide a lot of blood calcium (and a little vitamin D). However this also depresses vitamin D levels and the body's ability to absorb magnesium – catch 22. Dairy gives you high blood calcium, but low bone calcium.

Much work has been done on the effect of vitamin D with bones. For example, in 1991 Tufts University, Boston showed that vitamin D was essential for improving bone density and supplementation was important in the winter months. This work was confirmed in Lyon, France in 1992 where a group taking 800 IUs of vitamin D and 1.2 gms of calcium per day had 43 per cent less hip fractures and 32 per cent less other, non-vertebral fractures.

Sources
Sunlight on our skin is now thought to be the main 'source' of vitamin D. Whilst a little is found in dairy, the major source is fish liver oils and particularly cod liver oil. Plants contain very little vitamin D. Kidney or liver disease (and alcohol) depresses vitamin D levels, as do cholesterol-lowering drugs (e.g. statins), mineral oils, anticonvulsants and toxic chemicals in the environment (e.g. smog). Cadmium blocks vitamin D production whilst pantothenic acid helps make it. Night shift workers have lowered blood levels of vitamin D. Heavily tanned, or black people cannot make vitamin D through the process of sunlight in their skin.

RDA
The RDA was set at 5 to 10 micrograms (about 200 IUs) from that work over 50 years ago.

However, Dawson-Hughes (*American Journal of Clinical Nutrition* 1995: 61) has shown that at that level it has no effect on bone status at all.

Reinhold Veith PhD, University of Toronto, has concluded adults need five times this level (*American Journal of Clinical Nutrition* May 1999).

On a sunny day the body delivers about 10,000 IUs that makes a bit of a mockery of the official safety limit for supplementation of 2000 IUs. Veith proposed a level of 4,000–10,000 IUs per day and argued that toxicity doesn't start until about 40,000 IUs (*American Journal of Clinical Nutrition* 1999: 69). And Harvard Medical researchers totally agree with him.

Is that all?
Well now we come to the 'newer' discoveries.

Firstly vitamin D seems to help the body assimilate vitamin A and has a synergistic effect with both A and E.

Then came the finding that vitamin D stimulates the pancreas and helps in the production of insulin. In cases of vitamin D deficiency the body loses its ability to fully produce insulin.

Next, vitamin D was found to be crucial to the growth and maturation of the immune system white cells and thus people started to become interested in its effects on the immune system as a whole.

Vitamin D and cancer
Vitamin D plays multiple roles in the regulation of animals' metabolism; Boston University School of Medicine (Rahul Ray) showed that it has a regulatory effect on plasma membranes

affecting all sorts of carried hormones and chemicals, and also on gene transcription. They have conducted much work on vitamin D Nuclear Receptors (VDRs). Basically vitamin D is bound in plasma and on nuclear sites and is very much part of the **endocrine system**.

Epidemiology studies have argued that the levels of sunlight and cancer are inversely proportional. Studzinski and Moore (*Cancer Research* 1995: 55) talked about a 'belt' through America where there was less sunshine and 2–3 times higher rates of cancer.

But where cancer researchers were really turned on, was in the finding that vitamin D can regulate cell differentiation and proliferation.

For example, laboratory tests have shown that vitamin D inhibits the growth of the new blood vessels needed by tumours in order to satisfy their high metabolism (Shokravi et al Inv Cph 1995: 36).

Furthermore, cancer cells are undifferentiated – they act like foetal cells, being young and dividing rapidly and, as yet, not differentiated into lung cells, or liver cells or breast cells. Vitamin D can switch them over to be 'normal'. And right now drugs companies are trying to patent drugs to do this! (Why not just give people vitamin D?!)

Professor Michael Holick, an endocrinologist from The Boston School of Medicine has argued that 25 per cent of the women who die of breast cancer would not have even had a problem if they had maintained adequate levels of vitamin D throughout their lives.

Black people, who cannot photosynthesise vitamin D under their pigmented skins, are known to get more prostate cancers than caucasians and Gross (J Urol 1998) highlighted the use of vitamin D in the treatment of recurrent prostate cancer.

Vitamin D is claimed to greatly enhance radiotherapy effectiveness on breast cancer treatment (Mercola, June 2003) and vitamin D is known to inhibit the growth of pre-malignant cells in the lining of the colon and reduces cancer tumours (Somer). In May 2003 at the Howard Hughes Medical School they showed that vitamin D detoxifies a carcinogenic bile acid, Lithocholic acid, and confirmed that vitamin D can reduce polyps in the colon, which often ultimately turn into cancer tumours.

Holick is clear that vitamin D reduces the risk of breast, colon and ovarian cancers, and named 13 others (from bladder to kidney to stomach) that he thought vitamin D could affect.

In our interview with the two Professors Powles of the Royal Marsden, we were interested to note that they have been providing vitamin D to their cancer patients.

In summary
icon's view is that although sunshine can give rise to skin cancer, the record levels of this disease are being driven by oestrogen and oestrogen mimics pre-sensitising men and women to harmful rays. Sunshine is a crucially protective element to Caucasians because it causes the production of vitamin D in the body and this in turn, is hugely protective against cancer.

Meanwhile it is quite clear that more is being learned about vitamin D all the time and every reader would be well advised to supplement with a pure fish liver oil daily.

Worryingly, of course, EU directives have set RDAs for vitamins and levels for supplements which are often woefully inadequate. Recent research on vitamin D merely highlights the conflict that at the same time as the bureaucrats are clamping down, the scientists are just discovering how these essential ingredients really work, and at much higher levels than they 'permit'.

(e) Vitamin E
icon October 2003

Vitamin E consists of a group of fat-soluble compounds that fall into two subgroups.

The tocopherols – widely available in Europe.

The tocotrienols – not on the European approved list and thought to be actively 'weaker' (but see breast cancer below).

History
In 1922 researchers stumbled on the fact that rats fed wheat-germ and lettuce were restored to full reproductive health. Factor X was dubbed the fertility vitamin and in 1936 it was renamed vitamin E.

Overview
Vitamin E is a super vitamin – the ultimate free radical buster.

It helps prevent cell membranes, especially brain cells, blood cells and immune cells from oxidative attack. It literally stops the fat in them turning rancid. It is especially protective of both the B and T lymphocytes in the immune system.

It works as an antioxidant, particularly in the lungs, protecting against toxic attack and air pollution.

It protects against free radical damage throughout the body. Selenium helps its action.

It prevents the oxidative destruction of other vitamins such as Beta-carotene, C and A. Inorganic iron destroys its action.

It works synergistically with vitamin C and vitamin A.

And it has certain, and very clear anti-cancer benefits. It

appears, for example, to inhibit the growth of cancer cells at the local level.

Vitamin E and cancer: a summary

Stomach cancer – Italian research has linked low vitamin E levels with stomach cancer.

Cancers of mouth and throat – A study in 1992 by the NCI showed that regular usage of vitamin E cut these cancers by 50 per cent.

Lung cancer – A study in 1990 at Louisiana University Medical Centre showed people with lung cancer had significantly lower blood levels of vitamin E. This was confirmed by a study in 1991 at John Hopkins School USA. Again in 1991, a Finnish study amongst non-smoking men showed that men with the lowest blood levels of vitamin E were 3 times more likely to develop the cancer.

Breast cancer – In the Spring of 2002, *Life Extension* magazine published an article in which it reviewed 12 different studies on vitamin E. Its conclusion was that vitamin E (tocotrienol – but not tocopherol) reduced risk by as much as 60 per cent. Our own St Bartholomew's Hospital, London has also shown that women with breast cancer have lower blood serum levels of vitamin E (1992).

Cervical cancer – Albert Einstein College of Medicine, New York showed women with the most severe lesions had lowest levels of blood serum vitamin E. This was confirmed in Seattle where the highest blood serum levels reduced risk by two thirds.

Prostate cancer – The *Journal of the National Cancer Institute* (1998) showed that a Finnish study, whilst studying the vitamin E effects on smokers, spotted that amongst over 29,000 males the vitamin E study group had a 41 per cent decrease in prostate cancer over the placebo group. The protected group took 50 mgs of alpha-tocopherol per day for 5–8 years.

All cancers – Researchers at Tufts University in Boston (1990) showed that, in people over 60 years of age, a daily dose of 800 IUs of vitamin E significantly improved the immune system function.

Natural sources
Both plant and animal tissues contain vitamin E; however since it is fat-soluble the best animal sources tend to come with high fat!

Tocotrienol vitamin E is found in unrefined palm oil and corn oil; whilst vitamin E is generally found in sunflower seeds, almonds, soya and wheatgerm (best sources) plus green leafy vegetables, liver, egg yolk, fresh oily fish, nuts in general, pumpkin and sesame seeds, sweet potato, butter and whole grains.

Enemies
Smoking, inorganic iron, cholesterol reducing drugs, mineral oils and polyunsaturated fatty acids will all reduce levels of vitamin E in the blood serum. Breastfeeding, pregnancy and people of low fat diets also need supplementation. Overcooking, particularly of oils, destroys vitamin E content.

Are you getting enough?
Jon Baron, a nutritionist in the USA, argues that you should be taking all four tocopherol varieties, and all four tocotrienol varieties daily.

Major research studies use levels of up to 200 mgs (approx 280 IU's). Just to confuse you, International Units (IU's) are the measurement most commonly found on bottles of pills.

This compares to the Recommended Daily Allowance (RDA) of just 10 mgs. Clearly our governments haven't talked to our scientists, as the Optimum Daily Allowance can be up to 20 times higher than the RDA.

Indeed whilst 100 to 400 IU's is a favoured level for dietary supplementation, short term supplementation of 1000 IU's is not uncommon.

An even bigger problem is that it is very hard to 'eat' an Optimal Daily Allowance.

Even taking vitamin E rich foods and eating large volumes of them throughout the day only takes you to about 25–40 IU's. Up to 60 per cent of vitamin E is also expelled daily in the faeces, further worsening the issue.

So this really is a prime example for the anti-legislation argument.

If vitamin supplements are restricted to RDA levels (levels which are well below those used in successful research studies), and meanwhile we cannot get nearly enough from our food (largely because of soil depletion), then we will be far more likely to become ill.

There are simply too many research studies on vitamin E to argue against – it is a very well researched vitamin.

Do the EU really have any justifiable grounds objectively for limiting the sales of this vitamin to such small RDA doses?

(f) Vitamin K
Eat your greens!
icon March/April 2004

We're learning all the time
Worldwide only a handful of researchers study vitamin K, although it has been long known for its role in blood clotting. It is also involved in bone health. Now it is known to play a role in cancer.

The RDA is only 65 micrograms for women and 80 for men but this will have to be adjusted as it looks like vitamin K is nowhere near as abundant as was first thought.

Sarah Beth of Tufts University at Boston has looked into the vitamin in some detail. Analysing 2000 households, she discovered that whilst the over 60s are okay, the 18–44 age group just don't get enough, and not even the RDA.

Phylloquinone one form of vitamin K (vitamin K1) is found in some oils, especially soy bean oil and in dark leafy green vegetables such as spinach or broccoli. One serving of either of these two will provide four to five times the RDA

Hyrdogenation of oils produces another form of vitamin K and, whilst as much as 30 per cent of 18–44-year-olds intake comes from this form, it is far less biologically active than K, in the body.

Vitamin K controls the formation of coagulation factors in the body, from the plasma of the liver. And two bone matrix proteins are vitamin K dependent.

So vitamin K plays a part in two growing illnesses, heart disease and osteoporosis.

So what's it got to do with cancer?
Recent vitamin K research is quite clear. It has an anti-cancer effect and is useful in the treatment of many different types of cancer including liver, colon, stomach, leukaemia, lung and breast.

Here things get a little complicated as there are several forms of vitamin K, designated K1, K2, K3 and so on. K3 is a synthetic derivative, whilst K2 is a bacterially produced variant.

K1 can be taken with chemotherapy to improve its effectiveness. Yoshida et al, Tokyo Medical University, Int. of Oncology September 2003 have shown K2 has an in-vitro effect on lung cancer cells, squamous cells and adenocarcinomas. This follows work showing apoptosis with leukaemia cells. These researchers actually recommended K2 as "safe medicine without prominent adverse effects including bone marrow suppression". Levels up to 75 micrograms were used.

D W Lamson and S M Plaza of Bastyr University, Washington have showed that the natural vitamins K1 and K2 are just as effective as the synthetic K3 and work by oxidation and modification as anti-cancer agents. Both K1 and K2 "may act at the level of tyrosine kinases and phosphatases. They are affected by vitamin K, which can lead to cell cycle arrest and cell death". (*Alt. Med. Rev.* August 2003). They went on to show **that 6 out of 30 patients with liver cancer had their disease stabilised after taking vitamin K**. This could be extremely significant research.

To achieve the levels used in the test could be almost impossible by just eating green leafy vegetables and supplementation is essential. (Take with a meal, as vitamin K is fat-soluble.)

Vitamin K is not even toxic at 500 times the RDA so there are few problems with dosage. 2000 to 3000 micrograms is often the recommended level for prevention.

There has been quite a lot of comment about vitamin K intake for pregnant women as a way of minimising childhood leukaemia. However Fear et al (*BJC* 2003: 891) found no connection between the lack of vitamin K and this disease. Another study by Dr Koike at Tokyo University that vitamin K slows the spread of liver cancer. 59 per cent of patients treated with vitamin K were alive two years after the test started, whereas only 29 per cent of the control group were.

Dr Koike said that K3, the synthetic form, might be more effective than K1 and K2 as it has been shown to interfere with electron transfer in the cancer cell mitochondria. It is not permitted in Japan.

Summary
Yet again, just like vitamin D, we are only really at the start of our voyage of discovery on the biochemistry of vitamin K. Clearly vitamin K has an effect on the notoriously difficult to treat liver cancer and there is definitely something worth exploring here.

And as usual, our modern diets, lack of greens, broccoli and spinach put our young at higher risk. Again, as with vitamin D, RDAs have been set before the crucial biochemistry is fully understood. Yet again the politicians are at odds with scientists. Supplementation, if you can't eat well, may be advisable.

(g) Selenium
You simply cannot lack this mineral

icon December 2003

Selenium – antioxidant, detoxing agent and cancer protector?

Selenium is an adjunct to an enzyme called Glutathione Peroxidase, which metabolises hydroperoxidases (especially found in polyunsaturated fatty acids) – unstable molecules also called free radicals. These molecules have a free electron, which desperately wants to pull in another electron and doesn't mind where it steals it. Thus it is easier to think of free radicals as molecules with superglue-sticky ends that can rip things off healthy molecules leaving them 'short' and needing to attack others to fulfil their structure.

Selenium is a mineral we are only just learning about. It was not even discovered as an essential nutrient until 1979 and only in 1990 was an RDA recommended. Selenium is now known to work with vitamin E and Glutathione Peroxidase to help prevent the body's tissues from damage.

Selenium has two other effects that may well play a role against cancer. Firstly, it protects the body against the increasing problem of toxic metals, for example, mercury, copper and arsenic. This is particularly relevant in the case of mercury, which pollutes via local coastal fish, fillings in our teeth and vaccines. The FDA in the USA identified some four years ago that 83 of the 100 most common vaccines used mercury as the carrier – by asking nicely they have reduced this to 73!!

Secondly, selenium levels affect your hormones – in particular, the thyroid hormone, from which selenium removes the iodine. This has a 'knock-on' effect to all your hormones as mammals are in a state of homeostasis, where all their hormones are balanced – throw one out and they all go out.

Selenium works in conjunction with vitamin E – both must be present to correct a deficiency in the other. They appear to work synergistically, protecting cells and their membranes. Selenium also appears to have an anti-viral and anti-bacterial benefit.

Various studies have looked at the blood selenium levels of people from different parts of the globe and the conclusion is invariably that low selenium levels are linked to higher cancer rates.

In 1984 researchers at the University of Kuopio in Finland looked at 8000 women and men who were interviewed and blood samples stored. In the following years 128 men developed cancer. When their blood was compared to those without cancer it was found to be deficient in selenium – in fact those with the lowest levels were three times more likely to develop cancer. It was reported that this was especially true for cancers of the blood and colon.

A second study by universities all over the USA looked at 11,000 people across five years. Of the participants, 111 developed cancer and again their selenium levels were much lower than healthy people tested. In this research the cancers most noted were again those of the gastrointestinal tract, but also prostate cancer.

By contrast selenium does not appear to influence breast cancer rates – the Harvard Medical School study on 62,000 nurses was inconclusive.

Males appear to have a slightly greater selenium requirement. It is lost in the semen and concentrates in the testes and seminal ducts.

One of the most important cancer trials was undertaken by the Nutritional Prevention of Cancer Study Group ('Effects of Selenium Supplementation for Cancer Prevention in Patients with Carcinoma of the Skin' Larry Clark et al, *JAMA* 1996) and utilised a 0.5 g high-selenium brewers yeast tablet providing 200 mcg of selenium per day. 1312 patients participated. This study showed that there was no effect on skin cancers in the group taking selenium, but a 52 per cent reduction in total cancer mortality, a 17 per cent reduction in all cause mortality, a 37 per cent reduction in total cancer incidence, a 46 per cent reduction in lung cancer incidence, a 58 per cent reduction in colon cancer incidence and a 63 per cent reduction in prostate cancer incidence. And this is in a group of patients in the United States where selenium intake from the diet is approximately 2–3 times higher than that in the UK and Europe in general.

Much work has also been done with the population of China where there are both selenium rich areas and selenium deficient areas. Research there suggests that selenium has a 20 per cent positive effect on cancer risk. The Americans conducted research using three antioxidants, selenium plus two others (beta-carotene and vitamin E) and showed a 13 per cent decrease in cancer rates. Recently the French studied 17,000 people with a five-antioxidant mix. This contained 100 micrograms of selenium and cancer rates for men declined 31 per cent and deaths from cancer 37 per cent during the five-year test.

Currently Dr Margaret Rayman, from Surrey University, a world expert in selenium is involved in the Precise study. Given a five star rating by the Medical Research Council, this is a major European trial (involving 35,000 participants Europe-wide) investigating the effect of supplementation on cancer at different doses. Funding is an issue at £2 million but hopefully will be sorted out soon.

Recommended daily levels and supplementation
The RDA is around 55 micrograms. It is felt that levels around 200 micrograms are probably beneficial but above that there is concern. At 900 micrograms there is proven toxicity, which manifests itself in dermatitis, hair loss and diseased nails.

Selenium yeast is the form of selenium used in the recent and most encouraging cancer trials, although usually this is not a live yeast. Someone who has a massive yeast overgrowth problem might need to stay away from yeast for a while, but this should not affect everyone.

Selenium yeast provides selenium compounds similar to those found in cereals, so closely resembles a food, which is ideal for a food supplementation (approximately 50 per cent of the selenium compounds found in yeast comprise of selenomethionine). Selenomethionine is another organic form and, whilst inorganic forms such as selenite and selenate are not naturally found in foods, they have been found to produce higher levels of glutathione peroxidase quicker. This is only one selenium dependant enzyme in the body and there are 35 or more selenoproteins that have been identified to date which all rely on selenium for their function. Bioavailability studies have shown that the inorganic forms of selenium are less bioavailable than organic forms.

Eating the mineral?
Try Brazil nuts (preferably the ones you crack), wholemeal bread, sunflower seeds and pumpkin seeds, free-range eggs, skinless chicken breast, tuna fish, onions, wheatgerm, tomatoes and broccoli. There is even a selenium-enriched form of garlic, which is giving strong anti-cancer results.

(h) Zinc
It's still a mystery

icon March/April 2004

Heavy metal
Some writers refer to zinc as an antioxidant and although strictly speaking that is not true, it certainly helps other known antioxidants do their job.

The total body contains about two to three grams of zinc, a level second only to iron as a mineral. It is crucial for healthy growth in mammals.

The RDA is 15 mgs and symptoms of zinc deficiency are a reduced immune system, poor wound healing, susceptibility to infections, loss of taste, smell and appetite, hair loss and skin rashes.

Zinc will slow the greying of your hair, prevent white spots on your nails (a sign of deficiency) and it is crucial to a healthy prostate and a healthy sperm count in men.

An excess of dairy reduces the body's ability to absorb zinc. In turn, this will make children 'picky eaters' and reduce their appetites. So giving milk to kids is no food substitute – it worsens the situation when kids do not eat.

Alcoholics and people taking B6 need higher amounts of zinc.

Sources
Best sources are wheat germ, liver and oysters, followed a long way behind by pumpkin and sunflower seeds then nuts like pecan and brazils, steak and other meats.

The biggest problem in the Western world is that the process of refining wheat removes around 80 per cent of its zinc content.

Not surprisingly one UK government study found that zinc intakes for men and women were only 50–75 per cent of recommended levels.

Zinc is available as a supplement in sulphate, gluconate, picolinate and other forms all of which are well absorbed.

What does it do?
Zinc is involved everywhere in the body. It helps the action of vitamin C and is helped itself by vitamin A.

It is involved with many metabolic enzymes and is a constituent of the important antioxidant enzyme superoxide dismutase. Thus it plays a part in preventing the formation of free radicals and also of neutralising them.

It is capable of boosting the immune system and particularly the number of white cells in the bloodstream. Results from Belgium in 1981 showed that a group taking zinc supplements had significantly higher circulating white cells and antibodies to an infecting agent, than the control group.

Finally, one of zinc's most important functions is in the synthesis of both RNA and DNA. Somer (Harper Perennial 1995) coupled these last two points and concluded that therefore zinc must play a role in cancer prevention however, to date, no one has actually discovered it!

The fact is that where zinc is concerned the biochemistry of its action is still in its infancy. "The effects of zinc on the initiation and progression of cancer are not well established, although the negative effects of zinc deficiency on the immune system are clear" (M C Linder *Nutritional Biochemistry and Metabolism*, Elsevier Science Publishing, 1991).

There is a view that zinc, which is normally stored in a healthy prostate can be displaced by toxic heavy metals such as nickel and that these are implicated in prostate cancer. In a paper presented to the American Society for Cell Biology in 2001, it was reported that malignant prostate cells lose the ability to accumulate zinc. A healthy prostate has between 3 and 10 times more zinc than any other tissue, but a malignant prostate has very low levels. Fenn, Franklin and Costello of the Greenbaum Cancer Centre reported that high levels of zinc act as a brake on runaway prostate cell growth by increasing malignant cell death. Malignant cells' mitochondria lose the ability to utilise zinc, and then multiply uncontrollably. Zinc supplements triggered an enzyme called cytochrome C that caused apoptosis.

However to counter this, Leitzmann et al (Journal of the National Cancer Institute, July 2003) tracked 46,974 men from 1986 to 2000 and showed that men who consumed more than 100 mgs per day of zinc had just over twice the risk of prostate cancer, as did men who took supplemental zinc for 10 years or more!

Summary

The problem for everyone reading this piece is who to believe. Whilst it is clear that zinc plays a part in the cancer process, no one really knows what part. With prostate cancer, clearly taking too much may worsen your risk (too much being over 100 mgs per day, or too much may be every day – although the research did not quantify the level). Equally the level to cause apoptosis is not confirmed.

So it all remains a mystery for the time being.

(i) Magnesium
Missing magnesium

icon July/August 2004

Magnesium shortages abound in the West
In January a research study in the US showed that 40 per cent of Americans were deficient in magnesium. Blood plasma studies in the UK show similar shortages. But is it any surprise?

Firstly, a report in February 2004 by David Thomas, a mineralogist and fellow of the Geological Society, using the Government's own data showed that between 1940 and 1990 vegetables had lost over half their content of calcium and magnesium, while mineral levels in fruits fared little better. Findings were supported in the British Food Journal by Anne-Marie Mayer, a nutrition researcher at Cornell University, USA. She examined 20 fruits and 20 vegetables and found significant reductions in levels of calcium, magnesium, copper and sodium in vegetables and in magnesium, iron, copper and potassium in fruits.

Both researchers link the decline to intensive farming. They suggest that agricultural chemicals and a lack of crop rotation may be depriving plants of minerals.

Secondly, we are consuming too much dairy, and dairy consumption can depress magnesium levels in the body.

Finally, we eat less of the foods that have historically given us our magnesium. Foods like fresh nuts (for example, almonds), pulses (for example, lentils, broad beans, peas), green leaf vegetables, jacket potatoes (including the skins – don't microwave!), and the whole grains like millet, oats, buckwheat, wheat germ and complete brown rice. Refined grains lose 80-90 per cent of their magnesium content in the refining process. The only fruits with good levels of magnesium are bananas, mangoes and melons.

What does magnesium do?
The body contains about 25 gms of magnesium – it is everywhere. About 60 per cent is in the bones and teeth. The body needs magnesium for bone growth and to prevent tooth decay. Magnesium is needed for vitamin D synthesis and low vitamin D levels mean low calcium absorption. Worse vitamin D as we reported in **icon** February 2004, is increasingly known to be important in the fight against cancer.

So we have a vicious circle; too much calcium (over 1gm per day – or one good helping of green vegetables) depresses magnesium and vitamin D and means it is less likely to be taken up by the bones.

Magnesium is also crucial to a healthy liver, your organ of detoxification. It also activates over 300 enzymes throughout the body including some in the energy generation process in the power stations of all cells in the body.

As nutritionists like Gerson and Plaskett have shown, any inefficiency in the cellular power stations, in effect poisons the cell making it more acidic, less capable of using oxygen and generally producing less energy from the raw materials. Magnesium doesn't just work in some of the energy reactions, it activates a pump in cell membranes pushing sodium out of the cell and potassium into the cell. Too much sodium or too little potassium poisons the cell and sets up conditions of toxicity and the threat of cancer.

Magnesium works in muscles to help them relax (calcium helps them contract) and studies have shown that a higher magnesium intake may reduce the risk of heart disease and high blood pressure. A 1992 study at the Royal Leicester Infirmary showed a 24 per cent higher survival rate in a group of heart attack victims who were given magnesium by injection.

A good level of magnesium is also critical to a healthy liver. Alcohol and caffeine both cause the liver stress and deplete magnesium levels. In France or Italy being 'off colour' is usually put down to a 'liver crisis'. A few days off alcohol, a few more artichokes eaten, even certain magnesium rich mineral waters taken in preference to the usual tipple, soon has the patient recovering. In China too all patients have to show their tongue and eyes, both of which can show up an unhealthy liver.

The liver is of course our prime organ of detoxification and crucial to our health. In the UK we used to take Andrews Liver Salts, or drink or bathe in Epsom Salts to provide magnesium and aid detoxification. The French, Italians and the Chinese all understand its role in your daily health – 'une crise de foie' is a common Mediterranean concern. Why, the French even have a bottled water, Hepar, which has higher magnesium and makes healthy liver claims.

All cancer patients have an overworked liver as it tries to keep up with all the dead cells from radio and chemo, the harmful bacteria, maybe a virus or a parasite, the need to neutralise the lactic acid produced by cancer cells and on top of all this do its natural blood cleansing job. The liver may well be fatty, sugary, and even be 'clogged up' by gallstones. And if the liver does not work fully there is a knock-on effect to the whole immune system, throughout the body. Hence the need to detox, or use a liver cleanse, and ensure adequate levels of magnesium.

Diabetes, parathyroid problems, diuretics, alcohol consumption and diarrhoea/ sickness will all deplete your magnesium levels.

Change your diet; and think about supplementation. You simply cannot afford to be short of magnesium.

17 What else could help me?

Chris Woollams

(a) Glycoproteins and medicinal mushrooms

icon April 2003

Nobel Prizes

Four Nobel Prizes for Medicine in recent years (1994, 1999, 2000 and 2001) have been won with research on how cells communicate, and its importance to our health and well-being.

Whilst one of them was specifically concerned with the brain and how nerve cells communicate through chemicals with each other (Arvid Carlson et al 2000), the other three were concerned with communications to cells around the body and all had implications for cancer prevention and treatment.

In 1994 Gilman and Rodbell won for their discovery of 'G-proteins and the role of these in signal transduction in cells'. Basically they investigated how localised cells handle signal substances from glands, nerves and other tissues to make changes.

In 1999 Gunter Blobel and his team looked at how proteins have specific protein signals built into them so that they reach the correct destinations.

And by 2001 Hartwell, Hunt and Nurse had won for showing an understanding on the cellular messages involved in the cell cycle – its growth and division into two identical daughter cells – and how mistakes might result in a cancer development.

These protein messages often involve carbohydrate molecules, or sugars, and so a generic term Glycoproteins is the word coined for this hot topic.

A simple explanation
Glycoproteins are polysaccharides with attached proteins or peptides which seem to 'control' their activity. Polysaccharides are long ' link chains', each link being made of a simple glucose molecule. The only problem is that you must 'eat' them as you do not possess the enzymes to assimilate them in the body from glucose building blocks. You also do not have the enzymes to break them down.

Several aspects of glycoproteins are important.

Blobel sought to understand a genetic mystery. When your DNA string is read and the code says you should have blue eyes or blond hair, how does the message get to the right place?

As a foetus in the womb, each of us started out with a fused cell from our parents that multiplied at an incredibly rapid rate. But around day 42-46 something (largely thought to be a message from the pancreas) tells these cells, called stem cells, to turn into eye cells or hair cells, and to stop dividing so rapidly and instead to adopt a normal cell cycle.

The interest for cancer scientists is that cancer cells resemble stem cells and do not seem to have received the signal to differentiate. Blobel found that the messages sent out contained little 'postcodes' directing the message to the hair cells or the eye cells. Furthermore he discovered that these signals contain the ability to go through the cell membrane and so influence the mechanism of the cell inside.

Cell membranes – barriers to health?
Cell membranes, like all tissue, are largely made up of fats or lipids, protein and carbohydrate. If you think of each molecule as a pin, with a pinhead, alternately pointing in opposite direc-

tions but in a neat line, you will have a picture of a healthy membrane. Messages can thus slip in between the pins. It is the role of glycoproteins to encourage this 'neatness' and thus allow the messages through.

The problem comes when the pins are not in this neat format and are fused or at various angles, not allowing anything through. Worse sometimes modest amounts of carbohydrate are bonded to the membranes.

Where tumour cells have this carbohydrate, it is used to bind to other cells and cause them to turn rogue too, hence causing metastasis. Killer cells in your immune system look out for these carbohydrate bonded sites.

Blobel's work focused on what happens when there are errors in the signals, while Hartwell et al focused on what happens when the cell cycle goes haywire.

What this means to you and me
The need for healthy signalling and message flow has led to a focus on glycoproteins.

Professor Gilbon-Garber has shown, for example, that the invasive process of bacteria, viruses and indeed cancer cells which involves the above 'bonding' process to membranes, can be inhibited by glycoproteins in mother's milk.

Because these molecules (from mother's milk, saliva and semen) used in her experiments are all natural, no side effects occurred.

This has important implications. "Drugs" could be built on natural substances, with no side effects.

So where can I get them?

A number of naturally occurring substances have already been identified as having high glycoprotein content. Not surprisingly one was Medicinal Mushrooms. Reishi, Maitake, Cordyceps and Oyster mushrooms all have beta-glucon polysaccharide. Cancer Research UK reported recently that Japanese mushroom pickers have half the cancer rates of the rest of the population. (They obviously scrump!)

Other natural sources of these essential sugars are:

- aloe vera, noni juice,
- brans – slow cooked oatmeal, whole barley, brown rice,
- pectins – apples, pears and citrus fruit eaten whole,
- breast milk,
- arabinogalactins – found in wheat, leeks, carrots, radishes, pears, red wine, coconut meat, tomatoes, curcumin and echinacea, corn, psyllium, garlic.

The interesting factor is the universality of the discovery. All cells seem to positively respond to glycoproteins, whether they are human, yeast, plants and animals.

Even tiny amounts of these sugars – or lack of them – have a profound effect.

One integrated cancer expert we spoke to said that glycoproteins would be more important than all discoveries like vitamin C, B-17 and genistein added together!

There is one commercial product, Ambrotose, recommended by a number of complementary therapists. However, it is worth noting that you should ensure you incorporate the above foods into your diet. Despite all the Nobel Prizes, any supplements for glycoproteins are unlikely to be on the new EU approved lists, as the directive currently stands!

(b) MGN-3

icon July 2003

MGN-3 has become increasingly popular over the last four years. In the UK it has a trade name, BioBran.

Many of the integrated doctors recommend it as part of their regime.

It is a powerful immune stimulant, and is often recommended to keep white cell levels up when chemotherapy and radiotherapy are doing their worst. It is however quite expensive at about £10 per day, which can be significant if people are using it over several months.

MGN-3 is not technically 'only natural' although it is made by natural action on a natural product.

Daiwa Pharmaceutical first developed it in Japan over ten years ago and it is claimed to enhance the activity of the immune system without undesirable side effects.

There is in fact quite a lot of good clinical research to support the activity of BioBran MGN-3. All of it Japanese.

It has been well documented for many years, that certain large polysaccharide molecules, for example complex carbohydrates such as plant fibres, can stimulate the immune system.

Fibre in general has also been linked in research to the lowering of cholesterol, improved sugar metabolism and the reduction of intestinal toxicity.

Rice bran also has anti-viral properties and certain mushroom fibres, for example those of cordyceps, reishi and maiitake, have been shown to contain beta-glucan polysaccharides, which appear to enhance immune response. Cancer Research

UK reported their anti-cancer properties in 200. Unfortunately, plant fibres are mostly indigestible, and so these immune enhancing benefits remain mostly unrealised as the fibre passes through and out of the body.

However, if these rice bran polysaccharide molecules are partially broken down into hemicelluloses, of which the most powerful are the arabinoxylan compounds, the smaller molecules can pass into the bloodstream and the benefits are magnified. The mushroom enzymes are used to achieve this and the resulting blend of hemicellulose compounds from this process is called BioBran MGN-3.

The exact mechanism of immune stimulation is not known, though it appears to occur by increasing the body's production of natural cytokines, for example interferons, interleukins and tumour necrosis factors, which mediate interactions between cells. Apart from inhibiting replication of viruses and having an anticancer effect, cytokines increase the activity of white blood cells or lymphocytes, including B cells, T cells and especially NK (natural killer) cells.

These protector cells go through the body destroying virally or bacterially-infected cells, or abnormal cells such as cancer cells.

In its lifetime, a single NK cell can kill as many as 27 cancer cells, sticking to them and then injecting lethal chemicals into them, destroying them in less than five minutes.

Most of the research papers done on MGN-3 arabinoxylan compound, involve testing of NK cell activity.

So MGN-3 seems to offer a double whammy: namely improving white cell count and strength whilst having the ability to attack cancer cells directly.

Interestingly, research has shown that small units from acidophilus cell walls can also destroy cancer cells in vitro and the Chinese have spent a number of years working on a treatment called CHML, which involves taking small active portions of plant cell walls and either injecting them into a tumour's blood supply or directly into the tumour. In both cases the results are remarkable and the FDA has taken out an exclusive deal with the Chinese to develop the treatment. Could this be a chink in the pharmaceutical companies' domination of cancer cures in the twenty-first century?

(Biobran, MGN-3 is available from The Really Healthy Company via the **icon** offices on 01280 815166).

(c) Aloe Vera

icon June/July 2004

A Mesopotamian folk remedy!
Dr Lawrence Plaskett, vice-chair of the Nutritional Council in the UK has said only recently that, *"It is amazing in view of all the positive indications which exist for all the anti-cancer effects of Aloe Vera that no medical studies have been initiated in human cancer".* The US Department of Agriculture has however approved Aloe for the treatment of soft tissue cancers in animals (1992) as well as feline leukaemia; and Aloe is approved as an important component in European AIDS therapy where it has a powerful effect on the immune system and complements certain drug therapies.

Origins
Aloe's first recorded use was in Mesopotamia in about 1500 BC. It was then favoured by both Egyptians and Greeks for the immediate treatment of burns, cuts, wounds, infections and even 'parasites'.

Aloe is a member of the lily family belonging to the group Xeroids, and grows in dry regions of Africa, Asia, Europe and America. There are 200 varieties of which four have nutritional value, the most common variety being Aloe Barbendis Miller.

The usual debate is about the relative merits of the whole leaf or the gel. Some companies claim the inner leaf has the most benefits whilst others claim the outer leaf and rind are the crucial elements. Whatever the debate, Aloe is very well researched. In fact it has almost so many 'benefits' it is easy to feel many of these are overclaims – but they are not!

People in the West started drinking Aloe gel in the late 70's as brands became available, with claims for nutritional, skin care and even weight loss benefits. It can also alkalise the body.

However, recent years have seen biochemistry explain the various benefits of Aloe.

Active Compounds
What doesn't Aloe have? Over 200 active compounds have been recorded including vitamins, amino acids, minerals, enzymes, polysaccharides, fatty acids and more. For example:

Polysaccharides and Glycoproteins – We have covered this group of compounds before in **icon**. In 1994 Gilman and Rodbell won a Nobel Prize for showing how 'G-proteins' help cells send messages inside them. By 1999 Blobel had won one for showing how messages pass round the body and in 2001 Hartwell, Hunt and Nurse won one for showing how cell messages operate in growth, division and mistakes. Such signals can 'clean up' membranes and receptor site like the diabetes receptor site whilst others pass across membranes. Of particular importance is the way bacteria and viruses, for example, bond to locations on membranes. The latter is inhibited by glycoproteins and polysaccharides.

The most potent polysaccharide in Aloe is Acetylated Mannose or Acemannan, which is used in European AIDS treatment. Dr Akira Yagi and his team at Fukuyama have isolated a number of these **polysaccharide**, **phenolic** and **chromone** compounds and these are at the core of Aloe's anti-viral, anti-bacterial and immune boosting powers. Large polysaccharide molecules from Aloe have been shown to produce Tumour Necrosis Factor in the body, shutting off the blood supply to tumours. Others increase Interferon and macrophage production and T-cell quantity. But in cancer patients T-cells look for clear distinguishing areas on cells to sort the good from the bad and normally only one in a thousand T-cells can actively 'spot' a rogue cell. Aloe polysaccharides also appear to dramatically improve this ratio. So it is quality, not just quantity, that improves!

Anti-inflammatory benefits – There are a number of active compounds which reduce inflammation and can thus help in conditions from arthritis to wound repair, acne and insect bites. Fatty Acids, like **gamma-linoleic acid,** reduce inflammation, allergic reactions, blood platelet aggregation and improve wound healing. **Salicylic** acid is commonly found as aspirin and since 1982 Nobel Prize winner Sir John Vane's work on cellular environments we have known this can control excess prostaglandin production along with other negative factors. **Gibberlin, sterols** and the amino acids **phenylalanine** and **tryptophan** are also involved in anti-inflammatory processes and wound healing.

Other Benefits – Certain enzymes **(Bradykininases)** break down Bradykinin, which is a peptide substance causing increased vascular permeability. Aloe can help blood and lymph circulation. In wound healing Aloe doesn't just inhibit acute inflammation (like steroids) but stimulates fibroblast growth to improve wound healing and block the spread of infection (Dr Robert Davis, University of Pennsylvania). Its content of vitamin C, E and zinc will help this process. **Lignins** can help detoxify the blood and intestine by binding chemically to fats, and finally **anthraquinones** (aloin, aloe-emodin, barbaloin) are cathartic.

Sources – There seem almost too many suppliers of Aloe. Look for one that is organic and preservative free, contains no (artificial) sweeteners and has at least 90% juice content.

(d) Noni juice
icon July 2002

The Fruit of Life?
Morinda citrifolia, or Noni, is a knobbly fruit widespread in tropical countries from Tahiti through Asia and back to Hawaii. In the Caribbean it is called 'dog dumpling', but this sounds a lot less appetising! It can be eaten as the natural fruit but is more widely consumed in liquid form.

Noni contains a number of enzymes and alkaloids in quite large quantities. It would appear from several research studies to have four main benefits:

Firstly, it directly stimulates the immune system increasing the production of both B – and T – lymphocytes. Furthermore, Noni contains pro-Xeronine, which can be converted to Xeronine by natural enzymatic action in the body's tissues. Xeronine, produces a strong immune response to cancer cells in laboratory experiments.

Secondly, it appears to inhibit tumour development. Research conducted by Drs. Hirazumi and Furasawa at the Department of Pharmacology in the University of Hawaii, showed conclusively that the high polysaccharide content of Noni inhibits tumours in mice. Bromelain, an alkaloid and enzyme also found in pineapples and used in some dietary cancer therapies, is found in high levels in Noni and it is known to weaken the walls of cancer cells. The undoubted strength of Noni lies in this multi-polysaccharide, alkaloid and high phytochemical content. Dr D.L. Davis, the senior science advisor to the US Public Health Service is very clear that, "phytochemicals can take tumours and diffuse them".

Thirdly, Noni helps regulate cell function and cell regeneration. Dr Neil Solomon MD, PhD. conducted research with mice and showed that those fed Noni live 123% longer than normal. He believes this is due to Noni enhancing the body's natural healing processes and balancing the body's pH. Noni, in its concentrated form, provides a strong residue of alkaline ash in the body when consumed. This would serve most people well as their normal Western lifestyle and diet produces an acid body. A slightly alkaline pH is essential for the peak efficiency of the cellular biochemistry, and for the effective functioning of the immune system.

In a paper 'The Pharmacologically Active Ingredient of Noni', R.M. Heinicke of the University of Hawaii concludes that Xeronine protects and keeps the shape of protein molecules, which after passage into the cell, can be better used to make healthy tissue. Xeronine may also help protein molecules pass into cells by enlarging the membrane pores and, so the theory runs, the bigger the pores, the larger the protein molecules 'feeding' the cells and so the healthier they become. The juice must be drunk on an empty stomach as the pepsin and acid of the stomach will destroy Xeronine and pro-Xeronine. In fact, you should not eat anything for about two hours before and about half an hour after taking Noni.

Finally, Noni acts as an analgesic for headaches and as a healing agent for open wounds. Researchers in France have found that it is 75% as effective as morphine sulphate without the addictive side effects. In South East Asia, Noni is drunk to aid digestion and neutralise foreign bacteria in the stomach. And it is also used to put on cuts and wounds to speed up the healing process.

As an aside, there is a marketing war going on between Tahitian and Hawaiian Noni products! For example, *"Hawaiian Noni is 100% pure Noni while Tahitian Noni is a juice, not 100% pure, and made from concentrate"* (Hawaiian Noni web-site). To give the reader some feeling for the marketing fervour surrounding this product, there are almost 43,000 web sites for Noni!

There is one cloud on the horizon. The European Union, who

only recently decided to halt the sale of vitamins and minerals beyond those on a prescribed, agreed but very limited list is also looking to cut a plethora of 'health products'. One coming under the spotlight is Noni. The EEC wants to categorise these products as 'speciality foods' and these can only be sold if the producers give evidence on their benefits by submitting copious documentation.

Indeed Noni was banned for a period in 2002/3 since there was no safe upper limit set for the drink – but then a famous actor recently 'keeled over' and was rushed to hospital because he drank 14 pints of water in an evening – so presumably water will have to be banned while scientists deliberate over a safe upper limit for that!

(e) Chlorella
icon May/June 2004

The green life
Over 30,000 species of algae inhabit the earth, from microscopic blue green algae to giant kelp strands over 120 feet long. Microalgae or macroalgae, they are virtually all beneficial to humans.

Microalgae include blue-green algae such as spirulina and aphanizomenon and green algae such as chlorella and dunaliella.

Such algae are found always near a source of fresh water and represent the very first life forms on the earth, some 3.6 billion years ago.

Chlorella
Although there has been interest in algae as a food source for over a hundred years, only after the Second World War did this intensify as the Japanese, in particular, looked for ways to feed the nation. Algae can be produced on relatively barren land and at protein levels twenty times higher than soya beans.

Most algae have a structure like a virus, being very primitive with no nucleus but what differentiates chlorella is that it does have a nucleus which gives it so many of its 'extra properties' and in recent years this form has amplified the interest in algae and their benefits.

Thus, chlorella is a unique, single celled, fresh water algae. It is often dubbed, 'a pure food' or 'a whole food' because it contains vitamins, minerals, amino acids, enzymes and polysaccharides. Indeed almost everything you could want in a natural supplement!

- The vitamins are bio-chelated, which means they are wrapped up with amino acids and so the body assimilates them more readily.

- 18 key amino acids are present including all eight 'essential' amino acids.
- The enzymes include important digestive enzymes, often used in cancer treatments.
- The polysaccharides include mannose, arabinose, galactose, rhamnose and xylose, shown to be crucial in improving the quality of the immune system and the ability of cells to communicate, and hence white cells to 'recognise' rogue infiltrators.
- The DNA content of 3 per cent total volume and RNA of 0.2–0.3 per cent means it is nucleic acid rich – good for both growth and anti-ageing. (Dr Benjamin Frank, in his anti-ageing clinic, originally concluded sardines had the highest nucleic concentration but chlorella is ten times their level.)

Chlorella has ten times the beta-carotene of carrots and is rich in most B vitamins except folic acid, but particularly high in B-12 and so is excellent for vegetarians.

Apart from its benefit as a food, there are numerous studies, largely emanating from Japan (e.g. Sarkar 1994 or Hayatsu 1993 or Konishi 1990), which show chlorella to be a strong booster of the immune system. In particular chlorella will increase interferon production, which in turn stimulates macrophages (the 'digesters' of rogue cells) and T-lymphocytes (the identifiers of rogue cells). Not surprisingly several studies show that it combats infection (e.g. Konishi).

It has also been shown in Japanese research to promote growth in children and to be a strong aid to tissue healing.

Since chlorella is known to increase the white cell content of the body, it can prove an aid both during and after chemotherapy.

Following a paper by Waladkhani and Clemens in 1990 (Effects of dietary phytochemicals on cancer development) there has been increasing interest in the benefits of chlorophyll in general in the cancer fighting process. Algae, chlorophyll, chlorella and other such elements have all been tested, largely by the Russians, as agents for use with photodynamic therapy,.

The chlorophyll molecule is structurally very similar to the haemoglobin molecule, but whereas haemoglobin has iron at its centre, chlorophyll has magnesium. When light shines on chlorophyll it emits oxygen, the basic system of photosynthesis. These facts mean that firstly chlorophyll is relatively free to travel round the blood system non-toxically and secondly, in the presence of light, produces oxygen the very substance that cancer cells hate. Dr Bill Porter in Ireland is using chlorophyll agents in his Cytoluminescent Therapy – an updated version of Photodynamic Therapy. Porter feels that his 'agent' actually can start to work in the bloodstream even before he has used light sources to activate it.

Certainly, there is a lot of well-documented evidence from the Far East on the benefits of eating green vegetables for diseases such as colon cancer and for purifying the blood in general.

Chlorella is a particularly good detoxifying agent; it can help detox heavy metals, for example mercury, and pesticides from the body and is recommended in a number of detox diets. Indeed it is so powerful a detox agent that people taking their first 'doses' of chlorella may feel nausea, faint and lethargic.

This first form of life on earth will also aid your acidity/alkalinity balance.

Finally there is some indication that it increases the rate of multiplication of lactobacillus in the gut aiding, for example, your digestion and the production of biotin, a B vitamin helpful as an antioxidant.

You can take it daily and the best forms should never be freeze-dried. It should obviously have no additives or preservatives. Above all remember this is a **natural food**.

(f) Essiac
The medicine man's cure for cancer

icon August 2002

Essiac, which is sometimes called Cassie Tea, quite simply is a natural, herbal tea. Currently, it is unapproved for marketing in the University States and Canada.

However the Resperin Corporation, now owners of the formula, has a special agreement with the Canadian Health and Welfare department, which permits 'emergency releases of Essiac on compassionate grounds to cancer sufferers'.

Well does it work, or doesn't it?!

The original formula was given to Nurse Rene Caisse by a hospital patient who claimed her cancer had been healed some 20 years before by an Ontario Indian medicine man.

Cassie used the blend of herbs to treat patients for a number of years, setting up her own clinic in 1935 in Braceridge. Caisse's view was that it alleviated pain, and at the same time broke down nodular masses to form a more normal tissue. (Eventually the tumour would start to soften after an earlier hardening. Patients frequently reported a discharge of large amounts of pus and fleshly material as the tumour broke down.)

Her clinic was free, and by 1938 supporters tried to win government approval for her work, failing in parliament by three votes. Nine doctors had petitioned the Canadian federal health department as early as 1926 asking that Caisse be allowed to test her cancer remedy on a broad scale. In their signed petition they testified that the herbal treatment reduced tumour size and increased life expectancy.

Caisse's own view was that, if it doesn't actually cure cancer, it does afford significant relief. Whilst in Canada, Caisse treated her own 72-year-old mother with the tea under the supervision of Dr Roscoe Graham, consultant and specialist. The tea was administered 12 times a day for 10 days, and her mother lived to 90 years of age.

By 1942, without official approval and fearing arrest, Caisse shut her clinic, although she continued to treat patients at home. In 1959 at the age of 70 she went to the Breusch Medical Center in Massachusetts, where she treated cancer patients under the watchful eye of 18 doctors. Dr Charles Breusch, who treated President Kennedy amongst other members of New England's elite, reported in 1991 that he had been taking Caisse's formula since 1984 when he himself had cancer operations.

The original herbal ingredients were:

Burdock root: A well-known blood purifier that has been reported by Hungarian and Japanese scientists to decrease cell mutation and inhibit tumours. It has a reasonably high Selenium content.

Sheep sorrel: A traditional Indian remedy for everything from eczema to ringworm; it does have an effect in herpes, ulcers and cancer seemingly, by stimulating the endocrine system.

Slippery elm: Calcium, magnesium and vitamin rich, it had a healing effect on the lungs and internal organs. It also helps reduce acid ash in the body.

Indian rhubarb: Very cleansing to the liver and intestinal system. It also helps transport oxygen throughout the body and has an antibiotic and anti-yeast action and reduces inflammation. In 1980 studies showed that it also had a clear anti-tumour effect.

Whilst working with Dr Breusch between 1959 and 1978, Nurse

Caisse added four other herbs to the original formula. The new formula became Essiac, her name spelled backwards.

The four additions are:

Watercress: Strong antioxidant effects, contains bioflavonoids; it is a good source of vitamin C.

Blessed thistle: A blood purifier and immune booster.

Red clover: The herb of Hippocrates, the flowers are currently undergoing tests for breast cancer control.

Kelp: Like chlorophyll and spyrogina, kelp is a strong provider of natural minerals especially iron and calcium in an organic and easily assimilated form. Kelp is anti-bacterial, and sea vegetables in general help reduce acidity in the body, thus improving immune function.

Nurse Caisse recommended 12–13 cups of the infusion per day, although there are several reports of it being administered by injection. Shortly before she died she sold the 'secret' formula to the company Resperin.

Without proper clinical trials it is impossible to come to any definitive conclusion about Essiac and a degree of mythology has clouded some of the story.

What is apparent though is that the ingredients of Essiac, if nothing else, make it an excellent all round immune system booster and, whilst the specific anti-cancer claims may still need some hard supporting evidence, few people could argue with the proven track records of the ingredients. I can understand the banning of a cancer clinic without clinical trials, but hardly the banning of such a good all round cleanser and immune booster.

The medical authorities only play into the hands of the cynical and the 'alternative' health brigade when they refuse to conduct full and open clinical trials to clear up the outstanding issues once and for all.

(g) Hoxsey – the quack that cured cancer?

In 1988 the Office of Technology Assessment (OTA) of the United States Congress commissioned a report on the Hoxsey Therapy. It was the first federal agency to review the therapy and did it as part of a study into alternative cancer treatments. Patricia Spain Ward PhD, a medical historian from the University of Illinois, completed a background paper for Congress; this paper details the full story. Here is a summary:

Harry M Hoxsey (1901–1974) developed and practiced a cancer treatment. Since his death Mildred Nelson, his long-time nurse and assistant, has continued his work. In 1963 Hoxsey chose a site in Tijuana, where today stands the thriving Bio-Medical Centre, home of the therapy.

Hoxsey started life as a miner before turning to life as a healer in the 1920s. He believed that cancer was systemic – a disease of the whole body – and developed a herbal mixture to kill it off.

His first 'therapy' was in fact an external paste, made of antimony sulphide, zinc chloride, bloodroot and other occasional ingredients like arsenic sulphide, herbs and talc. With the help of Dr Frederick Mohs, a surgeon and the Dean of Wisconsin Medical School and several of its staff, he treated surface cancers that were then surgically removed with success. Hoxsey's 'red paste' and the experiments were written up extensively in the 1940s. Dr Mohs published in 1941 in the Archives of Surgery and in 1948 in the *Journal of the American Medical Association* (*JAMA*).

However the AMA attacked and attacked, even claiming that Hoxsey and Mohs had used different pastes. One report claimed that Hoxsey's active ingredient in the 1950s was arsenic, but it turned out the AMA was using an early 1920s paste! Hoxsey had developed a caustic treatment and was an ex-mining quack. Mohs was a doctor and a surgeon, and his treatment by contrast was acceptable. In fact both men were using sanguinarine, an alkaloid in bloodroot which has potent anti-tumour effects (Young 1967).

Worse, Hoxsey had an elixir for internal cancers. And he refused to tell people, especially the AMA, what was in it! In his autobiography in 1956 Hoxsey claimed his great-grandfather, a horse breeder, had cured his favourite stallion by giving him herbs from a particular field. Hoxsey Senior collected and mixed them but although he identified alfalfa, buckthorn, red clover and prickly ash he could not/did not name the others. Great-grandfather John had gone on to add yet more herbs and become a horse healer, and sometime human cancer healer too!

Harry Hoxsey's success as a healer, the wealth it created, and his refusal to divulge the exact ingredients of his elixir made him enemies in high places.

By 1950 the FDA used the courts to demand ingredient labelling and block interstate shipments. This forced Hoxsey to reveal all, and he detailed a core set of ingredients, with variant extras depending upon the individual and their type of cancer.

The basic solution was:

    Cascar (Rhamnus Purshiana)
    Potassium Iodide

The additions might include any of the following:

    Poke root (Phytolaeca Americana)
    Burdock root (Arctium lappa)
    Berberis root (Berberis vulgaris)
    Buckthorn bark (Rhamnus frangula)
    Stillingia root (Stillingia sylvatica)
    Prickly ash bark (Zanthoxylum Americanum)

Both the AMA and FDA dismissed the potion as "worthless, without any therapeutic merit in the treatment of cancer", and did not even analyse it.

In the *JAMA* 1954 the AMA insisted that "any intelligent physician could testify that all these substances were worthless". All Hoxsey's case histories at the subsequent FDA trial were dismissed as lacking in evidence and neither the FDA nor the NCI provided any detailed counter evidence or laboratory trials on cancer efficacy or otherwise. Commissioner Larrick warned Hoxsey publicly in 1956.

However recent literature fully supports the ingredients. For example:

Pokeweed – triggers the immune systems, increases lymphocytes and increases levels of immunoglobulin (Farnes 1964, Downing 1968).

Burdock – 'considerable anti-tumour activity' (Szeged University 1966), 'uniquely capable of reducing mutagenicity' (Morita et al 1984).

Burberry – anti-tumour activity (Hoshi et al 1976), contains lycbetaine, an anti-tumour substance (Owen 1976).

Buckthorn – anti-leukaemia substances; anthraquinone works against tumours (Kupchan 1976).

Even the least studied herbs, stillingia and prickly ash, have anti-inflammatory or anaesthetic properties and are used in European folk remedies.

An eminent US botanist, James Duke PhD of the United States Department of Agriculture, has confirmed that all of the Hoxsey herbs have known anti-cancer properties and have long been used by native American healers to treat cancers. Even as long ago as the 1850s, Dr J W Fell of the Middlesex Hospital was using bloodroot and zinc oxide directly onto malignant growths with great effect.

Hoxsey also had his 'converts'. The Assistant District Attorney of Dallas, Al Templeton, arrested Hoxsey almost 100 times until in 1939 his brother developed a cancer and was cured by Hoxsey. Templeton became Hoxsey's lawyer.

Esquire magazine sent journalist James Burke to Texas in 1939 to write a story 'on the quack'. He stayed six weeks, wrote 'The Quack Who Cures Cancer' and became his publicist!

In 1954 an independent team of ten US physicians made a two-day inspection of Hoxsey's clinic, then in Dallas, and concluded that he was 'successfully treating pathologically proven cases of cancer, both internal and external, without the use of surgery, radium or x-ray'.

But the fact is that still the FDA and AMA have not tested the therapy! Even in 1965 Morris Fishbein, former long term editor of *JAMA* and voice of American Medicine for 40 years referred to Hoxsey as a charlatan and talked of "ghouls and cancer quacks". Patricia Ward in her report to Congress quotes this sort of attitude as setting the "low level of discourse and the emotional rather than analytical tone". Hoxsey sued Fishbein – and won.

By 1976 the Cancer Chemotherapy National Services Center researching plants used in folklore, noted that they often had anti-cancer activity.

Hoxsey's clinics were shut down in the 1950s, when even a 1953 Federal Report to the Senate stated that the FDA, AMA and NCI had organised "a conspiracy" to suppress a fair and unbiased assessment of Hoxsey's methods (The Fitzgerald Report). At the time the Dallas clinic had 12,000 patients.

Today the Bio-Medical Center combines the flexible Hoxsey

formula with diet, vitamin and mineral supplements. Liquorice and red clover, used in Essiac and prominent in tests with breast cancer at Royal Marsden are frequent herbal additions. The clinic is outpatient only. You arrive, ideally with all your reports and tests, and they see you for a day or two. You leave with enough potions and medication to last three or more months.

Dietary advice is usually to avoid foods that conflict with the herbs; like pork, carbonated drinks, alcohol, vinegar and tomatoes. Supplements include immune stimulants, yeast tablets, vitamin C, calcium and laxatives. However the clinic does offer treatments like homeopathy and even chemotherapy.

External cancers like melanoma are frequently treated, as are cancers of the blood system. There are many case histories, though, for all cancers from breast to colon.

According to Nelson, about 80 per cent of patients seen at the clinic 'benefit substantially'. Steve Austin a naturopath from Oregon, followed 22 Hoxsey patients, and after five years eight were cancer free. Austin is now preparing a fuller study.

Ironically Hoxsey himself died of prostate cancer – and, yes, he did take his own therapy. In cancer treatments there are no guarantees.

(h) Hydrazine sulphate

To be published in a future issue of **icon**.

A goldmine in cancer treatment?
In the late 1960s Dr Joseph Gold had a flash of lateral thought. Instead of tackling the cancer cells, why not tackle the ultimate cause of death in patients undertaking chemotherapy, namely cachexia? Estimates vary but as many as three quarters of patients on chemotherapy may actually die from debilitation and weight loss rather then the actual cancer.

Cancer cells produce their energy in the absence of oxygen. They take in glucose and, by a short four-step process, manufacture some energy – but nowhere near as much as a healthy cell does with its twenty-six steps. The waste product from a cancer cell is very specific: lactic acid. It can only be broken down by the liver where, in turn, its end product is glucose. They are really rather clever, these cancer cells. They take over the host and use its own systems to generate their food supply, just as a parasite might do. This inefficient process, coupled with certain damaging effects of chemotherapy, can produce the debilitation and weight loss. The body is, after all, producing far less energy than normal, and the little it produces is feeding growing cancer cells!

Gold proposed hydrazine sulphate (HS) as this anti-debilitating agent because it could inhibit the gluconeogenic enzyme at the heart of the problem.

He then argued that if the tumour energy gain and the host energy loss (resulting from the cancer induced excessive gluconeogenesis) were actually interlinked, hydrazine sulphate could probably break the downward spiral and prevent the parasitic cancer cell being continually fed its favourite food.

Starting with rats and mice he showed that the above hypothesis was true. Without direct cytotoxicity, hydrazine sulphate seemed to amplify the effect of the chemotherapy yet appeared to have no side effects.

The politics begin
On 8 March 1976 congressman James Hanley requested a progress report on HS from the NCI. They provided an answer saying that clinical trials had taken place in Russia (Dr Michael Gershanovich) and no evidence of effect had occurred. In fact a few days later the actual report emerged from Russia saying the opposite! "Clinical observations enabled us to state a definite effect of HS in patients, when other measures failed" (Seits, Gershanovich et al Vopr Onkol 21, 45 1975). Indeed, because of the positive findings, the Russians actually enlarged the test!

By 1975, a phase II clinical trial from Russia using 'factually terminal' patients reported that 58 per cent demonstrated anti-cachexia response and 35 per cent anti-tumour response. The trial was then enlarged. A second pharmaceutical-sponsored study of 84 terminal patients produced responses of 59 per cent and 17 per cent respectively.

By 1979 the Soviet study was enlarged to 225 patients, with 65 per cent and 44 per cent responses respectively. This was reported in March 1979 (Proceedings of the American Association for Cancer Research).

Meanwhile the US authorities response was again nothing short of scandalous; with people recruited for trials dying within 11 days of the start, or no controls exerted over other drugs administered, often those which inhibit the action of Hydrazine Sulphate.

Finally in 1981 the American Cancer Society sponsored a double-blind, randomised, placebo controlled trial and by 1984 reported that in 38 patients with all manner of cancers, HS had shown activity. "Alteration of abnormal host metabolism could result in measurable clinical benefits, including weight improvement and stabilization" (Chlebowski, Heber, Richardson, Block, Cancer Research 33, 1984).

This breakthrough research should have put an end to the politics. It didn't. And it still continues today. Gold, who stayed silent throughout, has recently given a complete picture of it all – with an appendix of 78 peer group papers on the subject (The Truth About Hydrazine Sulphate: Dr Gold Speaks. www.hydrazinesulphate.org/). This 2004 paper is his first public comment on it all.

Activity
Hydrazine Sulphate is a low cost chemical and this may account for much of the politics. However it can be contaminated and so has to be supplied by a reputable dealer.

It is a monoamine oxidase inhibitor. It is incompatible with tranquilisers, barbiturates, alcohol and other central nervous system depressants. They can destroy its action. Also foods high in Tyramine, for example aged cheese or fermented products, are to be avoided.

Perhaps the most recent scandal belonged to the NCI who reviewed the product in 1994 (Journal of Clinical Oncology) and said, basically, that it didn't work. However they appear not to have been very strict in controlling the intake of the trial sample. Under direct orders from Congress a review showed that 94 per cent of the patients had taken benzodiazeprine or phenothiazine, 50 per cent on a long-term basis (Journal of Clinical Oncology, June 1995), thus wiping out the effect of the HS!

Probably two studies stand out. The Russian study above, and a study which subsequently corroborated it by Harbor, UCLA (Filov, Gershannnovich et al, Invest. New Drugs 13, 89-97 1995). If this were replicated in real life in Britain we could expect of every 100,000 late stage cancer patients treated, perhaps 50,000 would show measurable symptom improvement and 40,000 actually some regression. Surely this is not something to hide or belittle?

Side effects
Few are reported; sometimes tiredness, a little dizziness, pins and needles and occasional nausea. Usually though the patients claim a more positive outlook on life.

Latest developments
The Russians are still using HS to great effect. In Russia HS is called Sehydrin, and they have completed studies on all manner of cancers from lung to brain tumours (see http://scri.ngen.com).

I started looking into HS for my daughter who had a grade IV brain tumour. Of most relevance to her condition is a Russian study published in 1994. Patients with malignant brain tumours having chemotherapy and taking hydrazine sulphate had symptom response of 61 per cent and partial regression of 71 per cent, quite incredible findings given the *Lancet* paper of February 2004, which basically says that no Western brain tumour chemotherapy drug actually works!

Treatment
Dosage usually starts low and builds to 180gms maximum. It is recommended that you work with a doctor at all times on the treatment programme – a doctor with experience of using Hydrazine Sulphate.

Remember: no barbiturates, sedatives, tranquilisers, alcohol, anti-depressants.

And avoid all cheese, all fermented products, smoked fish and meats, and even Monosodium Glutamate (MSG).

(i) Coral calcium
icon March 2003

The Okinawans live an island life surrounded by coral reefs; they consume a little meat and fish, and large quantities of fruit and vegetables. However, their calorie consumption is restricted because they eat less rice than the Japanese. The coral provides them with wonderful supplies of organic minerals. The Okinawans have half the cancer rates of even the Japanese and a life expectancy of 81.2 years.

Coral calcium is a terrific alkaliser of the blood system and body overall, crucial in the fight against cancer. Calcium is not absorbed in great quantities by the body tissues unless there is magnesium and vitamin D present. High protein levels prevent absorption. Coral calcium contains high levels of organic calcium and magnesium plus other important minerals making them all easily assimilated by the body. Curiously after taking it for a month or so, particularly if combined with sensible diet and lifestyle, the body's alkalinity changes with the coral calcium but then self regulates as the coral calcium somehow seems to 'train' the system. Many cancer clinics recommend coral calcium.

Sadly in America the marketing has surpassed the product. Many websites claim it is some sort of cure for cancer. It may well re-alkalise the body, and in some cases where the cancer, for example, was caused by poor diet alone, this may help rebalance and detox the cells and body.

It is not a universal cancer 'cure' as some people might have us believe however. But a simple pH test, using what looks like a piece of schoolboy litmus paper under the tongue can show a reason to take coral calcium if the body is too acid.

(j) Mistletoe

icon November/December 2004

Mistletoe is a semi-parasitic plant that has been used for centuries in Europe to treat many human illnesses. Although the berries and the plant itself are poisonous, a whole variety of extracts has been prepared and these seem to avoid the toxicity and side effects.

The extracts are manufactured and marketed as injectable prescription drugs under a variety of names including Iscador, Isorel, Isucucin, Helixor, Plenosol and Eurixor. Some extracts are, in fact marketing under more than one name. Iscador, Isorel and Plenosol are sold as Iscar, Vysorel and Lektinol respectively. The chemical composition of the extract also depends on the host tree, and extract variants are prepared by tree type.

The extracts can be in aqueous solution or in solutions of water and alcohol. They may also be fermented.

The FDA has not yet approved mistletoe extracts and regards them as homeopathic drugs.

Why the interest?

Two components of mistletoe, lectins and viscotoxins, provide the probable active ingredients for the extracts, which have been shown to kill cancer cells *in vitro*, and to boost the immune system *in vitro* and *in viro*.

Viscotoxins are small proteins that appear to both kill certain cells by combining with their nucleic acids and stimulate the immune system. Lectins are larger and more complex molecules made of carbohydrate and protein (galactosides). They appear to be able to bind to the surface of immune cells and stimulate activity, in common with all glycoproteins. Glycoproteins improve intercellular recognition systems, activating natural killer cells/T cells and other white cells to produce interleukin 1 and 6, and also tumour killing factors. One study reviewed lectins' ability to release superoxide from certain white cells.

Does it work?
There have been over 30 European trials in mistletoe, none without a little bit of controversy. In 1994 a review of the trials found that there was insufficient evidence to recommend the use of mistletoe extracts in the treatment of cancer.

However a recent study (Maticek; Alternative Therapies in Health and Medicine May/June 2004) involving both randomised and non-randomised samples and 10,266 cancer patients changed all that.

A continuous recruitment of patients between 1973 and 1988 in Germany for the study based at the Institute for Preventative Medicine, United Nations, Heidelberg matched people treated with Iscador and those without with strict control of age, sex, tumour type, year of diagnosis, chemotherapy etc. A further follow up in 1998 reviewed survival times.

Both test groups showed an increased survival time of 39 per cent for those taking Iscador. Those who continued to use Iscador on a long term basis saw a doubling of survival time. By contrast, short usage times seem to provide little effect, possibly since stimulation of the immune system requires time.

Another study with patients having malignant melanoma is ongoing.

Treatment
Iscador is given as subcutaneous injection 2-3 times per week. Side effect are relatively mild and include a slight irritation or reddening around the injection site. There may be a rise in patient temperature.

A variety of cancers have been studied; from breast to brain tumours; from pancreatic to bladder cancer.

(j) Carctol

icon June 2003

Healing Herbs from India

Carctol is a combination of natural Indian herbs, for people with cancer and those wishing to prevent it. The herbs are recognised as having medicinal value in India, and several of them are recognised as such in the UK. So, although it has not been through the official licensing process in the UK (primarily because of the huge costs required), it is nevertheless classified as a UK medicine and can be prescribed by doctors over here.

Carctol is comprised of the seeds, roots and leaves of eight Ayurvedic Indian herbs. Volumes in descending proportions per capsule are:

Blepharis Edulis	-	200 mg
Piper Cubeba Linn	-	120 mg
Smilax China Linn	-	80 mg
Ammani Vesicatoria	-	20 mg
Hemidesmus Indicus	-	20 mg
Lepidium Sativum Linn	-	20 mg
Rheumemodi Wall	-	20 mg
Tribulus Terrestris	-	20 mg

The product is reported to be completely non-toxic and has been tested in both India (Institute of Medical Sciences) and London (Lyne, Martin and Radford).

Carctol would appear to have several benefits:

The web site says clearly that "Carctol is a herbal compound containing only rare, natural and indigenous Indian herbs mixed together with proportional strength to treat and heal all types of cancer" (sic). Treat and heal is a pretty strong claim!

The claim is then backed up by charts showing 1900 cases of

all types of cancer with groups who were 80-100 per cent symptom free ranging from about 30 per cent (oesophageal) down to 3 per cent (lymphoma).

The Daily Telegraph recently covered the story of Gwen Garner, a lady of advancing years, who had both a primary bladder cancer and a secondary pancreatic cancer. Being told there was nothing more the doctors could do, she went on a course of Carctol. Within 6 months the pancreatic cancer growth had stopped; the original bladder cancer disappeared.

The product is supposedly excellent when used during radiotherapy and chemotherapy, preventing patients becoming neutropenic (i.e. there is no compromise of white cells). This would give your body more of a "fighting chance". The oncology unit of Strongbrook Hospital, New York reports Carctol as a positive factor in the health of a two-year-old with cancer. She had no negatives during chemotherapy and even put on weight.

Nowhere does the information suggest how these eight herbs work. One UK doctor I know is prescribing it and she says that litmus paper tests on the tongue show the patient's system progressively going from acid to alkaline. Of course, this could be excellent as alkalinity is essential for proper cell metabolism and a strong immune response. But then the proponents of Carctol also demand a strict non-acid diet regime.

Simultaneously with Carctol, a vegetarian diet is recommended. As a minimum patients are advised not to eat 'acid foods' like unripe fruits, tomatoes, vinegar or oranges. Carctol works best with a good digestive system.

Normally one capsule is taken four times per day, but a maximum of eight is not unusual. Pre-boiled and cooled water is recommended, not tap water.

The effect is supposed to be slow and steady. A two-month trial

What else could help me?

is the minimum essential period, but more normally a six-month period is recommended with follow up periods.

Carctol is only available on prescription but apparently it makes a significant difference to those cancer patients on chemotherapy.

Ayurveda means "The science of life" and Indian medicine starts with the premise that a living creature is composed of soul, mind and body. Many herbs have been widely used for 4,000 years; the willow tree is a natural analgesic, and Neem, a tree has so many benefits it is often described as the "Village Pharmacy". It is anti-viral, anti-fungal, antiseptic and anti-inflammatory. Presumably it is also anti-EU?

18 Can Candida cause cancer?

Chris Woollams with Gerald Green

icon June 2003

I have a wonderful job. I meet so many interesting people, so many experts all on the same mission – helping people beat cancer. One minute it's Charlotte Gerson, then Dr Contreras. I may get a complex soon though; none of Britain's top orthodox doctors ever seem to ring me up to tell me of their latest work, which is very sad because **icon** now goes out to cancer patients in Britain's top oncology units every month.

One gentleman, with whom I have been corresponding, is Gerald Green, a medical herbalist and immunologist in Bexhill, Sussex. His grandfather, Professor Fritz Häber (1868–1934), won a Nobel Prize and was one of Germany's finest scientists – he worked out how to fix nitrogen, leading to fertilisers and bombs.

Energy and investigative endurance clearly run in the family. Gerald has devoted a large part of his life to studying 'Candida'.

It is estimated that 70 per cent of the British population have a yeast infection. The primary cause of this is our love of antibiotics. Swollen glands? Take antibiotics. Tonsillitis? Take antibiotics. Are you allergic to antibiotics? If the answer is 'no', that's fine. Antibiotics have no side effects.

Who says?

Friendly bacteria
Apart from a minor problem that they may well be toxic to brain

cells (Drs Goldman and Klatz, US), antibiotics kill **all** bacteria in the body, including the ones you need; the friendly ones in the gut. Acidophilus is on the supermarket shelves; you are urged to take it, but the damage may be already done. Acidophilus, for example, is known to keep Helicobacter pylori in check. If it doesn't because it has been killed off, Helicobacter pylori will embed itself in the mucous of the stomach lining and can then lead to ulcers and cancer.

The friendly bacteria in the gut perform a number of functions. They are the first line of the immune defence system; they produce useful vitamins like biotin, also helpful to the immune system and cellular health, they work with bile acids to extract and help you absorb the maximum level of minerals from your digested food and American research recently showed something amazing. Bits of their cell walls can kill cancer cells *in vitro*.

When they are not performing all these extremely useful functions they feed, especially when your stomach and intestines are at rest. At night their favourite food is yeasts and microbes.

It is not just antibiotics that harm the 'friendlies' – chlorinated tap water and acid bodies caused by stress and poor diet can eliminate them in just a few days, so you are wise to take a daily probiotic. The latest concern is that the new ubiquitous statins also cause their downfall.

Candida – out of control
Once out of control candida changes from the friendly useful yeast it was, into a very unfriendly parasitic fungus that can get to any part of the body and especially the vascular system. Once in the blood stream it is 'looking' for its favourite food, sugar – the patient's blood sugar which it ingests and converts into alcohol, turning the body into a sort of 'brewery'. This brings about the terrible fatigue all cancer patients have as their energy giving blood sugar is 'fodder' namely alcohol. The tumours then, in a chain of events, convert the alcohol into the

sweet smelling chemical athenol, the very smell Macmillan nurses often smell in a cancer patient's last weeks.

Diet
It is easy to see how yeasts have taken a hold in the Western world.

The USA and UK diets are simply weak in the foods that keep yeasts under control. A friend used to live in Thailand, a country with a trillion such microbes lounging on every street corner, but the Thai staples of coconut (caprylic acid), garlic, chillies and bee propolis are all natural controllers of yeasts. In the Mediterranean garlic, fennel and chillies do the job; in the Indian region it is Neem and garlic plus a host of spices; in the Caribbean it is nutmeg and cinnamon – the latter can even kill yeasts in your bloodstream. Our diets merely help to propagate yeasts and fungi. High sugar drinks, snacks, fast food, alcohol, refined wheat, indeed any high glycaemic food, feed the yeasts. And we live in high glycaemic land in the West.

A cause of cancer
I like Gerald Green. Of course, I'm biased. I always like people who share my views and we seem to have two views in common.

1. Candida is a part of the cause of most, if not all cancers.

2. Doctors rarely, if ever, stop to think about candida or parasite infection. And as a result their medicines only treat part of the cancer equation. In other walks of life it would be called: 'Neglect'. There, I've said it. (All the more odd, though, when even the WHO says 25 per cent of cancers are caused by infection).

I recently went to a cancer clinic in the USA, and to the Dove Clinic in the UK. At both I talked to the nurses. They were unanimous. **Every cancer patient they see, man or woman, has bad candida.** Whether it is breast cancer or prostate cancer. (It is most definitely true for my daughter with her brain tumour too.)

The problem is that these yeasts get everywhere. Whilst they might start off in your gut, they soon pass into the bloodstream and then, like Alien, they are loose in the mother ship. And they make an 'alcohol' as a by-product of their very existence which recycled becomes glucose, the perfect food for cancer cells.

Cancer treatments make matters worse!
To repeat: 'cancer treatments make matters worse!' Steroids and chemotherapy, for example, both heighten the effect of the yeasts, worsening the cancer cell feeding. It's like throwing babies to the sharks.

Take action
So back to the expert Mr Green. (And he is an expert. I have seen the letters he receives from hospitals and microbiology units saying he knows more than they do.) He believes even terminal cancer patients can be saved if the root cause is candida. And his favoured action is to use the herb 'wormwood' in conjunction with a rigorous diet. Gerald writes, "It is vitally important to kill candida and so break up the negative chain of events caused by candida. Wormwood has a unique triple action:

(i) namely to enhance the immune system by destroying its ball and chain candida;
(ii) so, as said, starve the tumours of their 'life blood' namely alcohol created by candida's demise;
(iii) while finally in the triple whammy, the live oxygen ions in the wormwood destroy the high iron ion content of the cancer tumour, in exactly the same way it destroys the also high iron ion content of the malaria parasite which led me to cracking this cancer issue". Indeed Professor's Lai and Singh at the University of Washington have reported on the use of wormwood to treat breast cancer cells. All such cells died within 16 hours (Life Sciences 70:1 Nov 2001). They

use artemisinin, a compound derived from the plant artemesia annue, or wormwood, used by the Chinese to combat malaria. (And recently approved by the anti-malaria Help agencies in Africa).

He believes you must **eliminate the following from your diet, immediately.**

All cows milk products:	cheese, yoghurt, whey. And all cow's milk derivatives which are everywhere in processed food.
Yeast products:	alcohol, bread, Marmite, Oxo, Bovril, vinegars, mushrooms, processed and smoked fish and meats.
All sugar products:	honey, fructose, lactose, glucose, dextrose and sweeteners like Nutrisweet and Canderel.
Nearly all fruit:	overripe fruits are full of sugar and yeasts. Plus vegetables like courgettes, pumpkin, squash, marrow.
High sugar root vegetables:	carrots, parsnips, sweet potatoes, beetroots, (maximum 1 potato per day).

Personally, I would add all high glycaemic foods to this list, e.g. refined wheat, rice, pasta, fizzy soft drinks, fruit juices and squash, biscuits, pastries, pieces, corn. Gerald mentions most of these too in his diet and he suggests you avoid all pulses, processed meats, high salt foods and hydrogenated vegetable oils too.

Below you will find his list of Good Food Choices. His sweetener of choice is Stevia, a herb one hundred times sweeter than sugar and also a natural anti-fungal agent. However it is not available for sale in the UK, you will have to buy it in the USA.

He recommends astragalus and echinacea plus 1 gm vitamin C daily to boost the immune system.

Good food choices
Eat plenty of the following foods:

Alfalfa sprouts
Bean sprouts
Bell peppers (sweet peppers)
Bok choy
Broccoli
Brussel sprouts
Cabbage
Cauliflower
Celery
Cucumber
Endive
Fennel
Garlic
Green beans
Hot chilli peppers

Kale
Lettuce
Onions
Parsley
Radishes
Spring onions
Spinach
Swiss chard
Turnips
Yellow beans
Granose sunflower margarine
Tomor kosher margarine
(both these margarines should be available at your local health food shop)

Fats (in moderation):
Avocado oil
Fish oil
Flaxseed oil
Grapeseed oil
Hemp oil
Mayonnaise
Monounsaturated fats
Olive oil
Primrose oil

Fluids
Try to drink 8 glasses of water each day.
Herbal teas are acceptable

Free range eggs
Fresh fish and seafood
Pork, lamb, veal
Poultry: chicken, turkey (particularly skinless white meat)
Game
Tofu
Quorn
Soy milk/cheeses (in moderation)
Rice milk
Sheep's milk/cheeses (dilute sheep's milk 50/50 with water and it will taste the same as cow's milk)
Goat's milk/cheeses

Culinary herbs and spices

Personally I would add that garlic, caprylic acid, oregano and Pau d'Arco are all excellent yeast raiders. His favoured natural destroyer is wormwood, which he says may only need a few days to achieve the desired effect. I always believe fish oils are a good supplement too.

However, you should note that the result is not the eradication of yeasts, but merely putting them into an inert and dormant state as spores. A week of binge drinking or sugary foods will soon have them thriving again.

Sure signs of yeast infection are wind after meals, a swollen stomach, yellow toe nails, thrush in women. Athlete's foot or spots in the hair behind the ear are external signs.

It is estimated that 70 per cent of Britains and Americans may have yeast infections, a truly Western disease.

The last word I leave to Mr Green. "The only difficulty in treating cancer is to keep the patient (especially males) on the anti-candida diet but this sadly is universally rubbished by 98% of the medical profession. Obviously with the doctors rubbishing all of these diets, their advice all but ensures the patient's demise".

However it is important to note that in the April 1993 magazine 'Contemporary Oncology', a peer reviewed cancer magazine in the USA, an article on the subject stated that, 'Cancer patients undergoing radio or chemotherapy often finally succumbed, not to cancer, but to an infestation of *candida albicans.*'

19 Things that go bump in the night

A summary and checklist for parasite avoidance in the body

Chris Woollams

icon November 2003 Centrefold

Few GPs will ever tell you that the cause of your illness is a parasite. And certainly none would ever be so 'trivial' as to tell you a parasite was the cause of your cancer.

But yeast infections like candida or fungal infections, microbes, amoeba, tapeworms and flukes are all parasites. And the fact that GPs never even test for these inhabitants is tantamount to negligence.

1. "I can't have a parasite!" Think again. You've eaten imported fruit, you've been abroad, had ice in your drinks, you've tried sushi, smoked or marinated fish. You've eaten undercooked pork. You could have threadworms from the soil.

2. The incidence of liver fluke in British livestock has quadrupled since 1997. Some microscopic parasites are immune to chlorine and have been shown to arrive in tap water in the USA.

3. It is estimated that at least 20 per cent of cancer patients have a parasite. Even the WHO (World Health Organisation) say that 25 per cent of cancers are caused by 'infection'.

4. BUT – yeasts, amoeba, fungi and microbes are parasites too. Normally your good intestinal flora – the friendly bacteria – feed off them at night.

5. What if the good guys are not there? Prescribed antibiotics, antibiotics in foods, steroids, cortisone, chemotherapy drugs, stress, nicotine, an acid body and over chlorinated water can kill off the good guys. Even GM food is apparently a threat.

6. Whilst fungal infection of the body may show up as yellow toenails, or thrush in women, more general symptoms include feeling bloated after meals, wind, irregular bowel movements, sudden fatigue, throat problems, a hangover when you didn't drink, mouth ulcers, allergies.

7. 70 per cent of men and women in the West have yeast or fungal excess in their bodies.

8. Specialist integrated cancer clinics in the USA and UK are clear. Every patient has a parasite – at minimum candida. 'Contemporary Oncology' (April 1993) said "Cancer patients undergoing radio or chemo often finally succumbed, not to cancer, but to *candida albicans* infestation."

9. All parasites deprive you of nutrients; all parasites produce toxins and/or alcohol, which feeds cancer cells directly.

10. How can you tell if you are infected? Go and see a homeopath for a Vega or BEST test. Have a stool test. Americans are far more conscious of this problem than the British – many Americans check every six months.

11. How do you remove the problem? Seven steps – **starve** the parasite, **kill** the parasite, **oxygenate** your blood, **alkalise** and **boost your immune system, building up the good guys, detox**.

12. **Starve** – cut out all cow's milk products; yeast products (alcohol, bread, marmite, Oxo, vinegars, mushrooms); all sugars and high glycaemic foods (like fizzy soft drinks and refined wheat); all sweet fruits (especially citrus) and cucumbers, marrows, squash; high sugar root vegetables (carrots, beetroot, parsnips).

13. **Kill** – wormwood, caprylic acid (coconut), Pau d'Arco, Neem, garlic, oregano, black walnut, clove, cinnamon (made as a drink from fresh sticks), fennel, bee propolis and hot chillies all work. (Look at the protective diets of hot climates.) Neways para-free is an anti-parasite herbal product taken over 2 months and effective with many parasites.

14. **Oxygenate** – yeasts and fungi thrive in anaerobic conditions. Like cancer cells, they hate oxygen. Exercise, learn to breathe, create an oxygen-rich body.

15. **Alkalise** – cut sodium, concentrate on potassium and magnesium foods e.g. lentils, nuts, bananas, apples, green leaf vegetables.

16. **Boost your immune system**; Vitamin C, beta-carotene, vitamin E, zinc and selenium. Fish oils with added A and D help gastro-intestinal deficiencies. Essiac, astragalus and echinacea all boost immunity and work against fungi. Take a good multi-mineral supplement too. And B vitamins.

17. **Build the good guys** – take probiotic supplements, eat live foods. Normally you have over 300 types of good guys weighing 1$\frac{1}{2}$ lbs in your gut.

18. Replace all sugars with Stevia – it is a sweetener, which is also anti-fungal and anti-parasitic. (You'll have to buy it in the USA).

19. Many fungi don't leave, they just become dormant spores. Don't let them come back to life. Stick to your diet.

20. **Detox** – use psyllium, Epsom salts, puri-tea (Neways) or even have colonic irrigation – it's a quick way to remove the dead cells.

20 Testing times

(a) Vega testing

Dr John Millward

icon December 2003

We are constantly reminded that our National Health Service (NHS) is failing to cope with the ever-increasing numbers of patients who are suffering from cancer and other chronic illnesses. Chronic illness after the age of 40 years is now the norm. Criticism of the NHS, although justified, is counterproductive unless it can lead to a radical new approach to the treatment of disease. The media constantly reminds us that we have a third world health service and that it compares badly with our continental neighbours. Many people would suggest that the German model of health care is not only better than our own, but that it could be a good example for this country to follow. However I suspect that most people have no detailed knowledge the German system, except that it can spare German doctors who come to this country and help reduce our surgical waiting lists.

Germany has adopted a fundamentally different approach to health care. There has evolved a holistic approach because German GPs are required to offer patients alternative medical treatments if conventional medicine doesn't work within a specified period of time. This has had two consequences. Firstly many German GPs themselves now offer alternative medicine. Secondly hospital consultants are prepared to accept alternative medical findings from both medically qualified as well as non-medical practitioners.

This holistic approach demands that equal emphasis is placed upon research into both conventional and alternative treatments. The discovery of homoeopathy is attributed to a German doctor. In England the few NHS homoeopathic hospitals still practice this original form of treatment, which is known as classical homeopathy. However other countries, principally Germany, have developed newer and more powerful remedies that are known as complex and resonance homeopathies. Also a variety of instruments have been developed to aid alternative practitioners. Many of these instruments magnify the subtle electrical currents that flow between the various parts of both individual cells and organs. It is now possible to use these instruments to assess the function of the various organs of the body and how both illness and treatment can affect them. American industry has realised the enormous potential of this approach to medicine and is rapidly catching up with the German technologies. In the USA this has led to increasing numbers of alternative practitioners, but as yet there has been little interest shown in combining both forms of medicine under the umbrella of qualified doctors. However in the UK the official attitude still discourages alternative medicine, its instruments and the newer forms of homeopathy.

Vega of Germany is an engineering company with a world-wide reputation for producing high quality measuring instruments. For many years it has also been involved in the research and production of measuring instruments for use in alternative medicine. It now produces a variety of models. There is a small portable version that relies upon the use of various test ampoules. The newer larger computerised version allows the practitioner to perform many more tests in a comparatively short time. By using the Vega, or similar, machine this enables an alternative practitioner to reach a conclusion within 30 minutes. This must be compared with the much slower and more expensive system of investigation that has been adopted by conventional medicine. This computerised machine is called the Vega Expert and the rest of this article refers to its use. Vega also produces a variety of more complex measuring and treatment machines.

In this country the name Vega has been associated with a number of bad news stories. This has been largely the result of unqualified people claiming to diagnose allergies and mineral/vitamin deficiencies. There is an interesting parallel between the Vega machines and the humble stethoscope. Anyone can buy a stethoscope, pretend to be a doctor, and then pretend to make a medical diagnosis. Heart specialists have to undergo many years of training before they can claim to make an accurate diagnosis using a stethoscope.

The Vega machines work by involving the patient in an electrical circuit. A baton is held in one of the patient's hands and the circuit completed by applying a stylus (like a ballpoint pen) to the opposite hand or foot. The process is non-invasive and painless. Is it easy to operate? Any doctor, dentist or nurse could learn to use it in a very short time. With practice comes expertise and a knowledge of the various alternative remedies. If it were a difficult technique there wouldn't be 14,000 to 20,000 of these machines in German doctors' and dentists' surgeries.

The Vega machine can be used for both diagnosis and treatment. Knowledge of basic anatomy and physiology is needed to help with making a diagnosis. Then the effectiveness and safety of any proposed treatments can be assessed. Therefore the range of knowledge possessed by the operator is the only limit to the range of treatments on offer to patients. I have found that the machine yields answers that make pathology become alive and therefore dispenses with the need to make vague or misleading diagnoses. After 30 minutes, or less, the operator is in possession of sufficient knowledge to make one of three choices. Firstly there may be the need to refer the patient on to another qualified practitioner for further advice and investigation. Secondly the patient could be offered conventional treatment, or thirdly alternative therapy.

So how does this machine operate? Like any machine it has to be calibrated and an initial test to determine if the patient is either healthy or not functioning properly. Because the machines are based upon the Chinese principle of energy and meridians it is possible to tell if the patients Yang and Yin are equally balanced. These two energies should be equally balanced. If there is too much Yang then the patient is hyperactive. If there is too little Yang then the patient is under active and fatigued.

There are two screening tests that can provide a variety of clues that can lead to more detailed tests and an eventual diagnosis. It is possible to discover if the patient is suffering from stress, is depressed or suffering from another mental illnesses. Surprisingly, despite widespread publicity, stress is rarely found. The diagnosis of stress is made upon personal opinions and there are no conventional tests to confirm this diagnosis. Viral, bacterial and fungal infections are shown in the screening test. It is important to distinguish between various infections because resonance homeopathic remedies are capable of destroying viruses. Although vaccine damage is denied in this country, it is accepted, diagnosed and treated on the continent. Consequently the machine has a screening test that not only demonstrates the presence of any vaccine damage, but which vaccine is responsible for that damage. Deficiencies of hormones, enzymes, minerals and vitamins can be highlighted. Tumours, if present, can be classified as benign, pre-malignant and cancerous. It is possible to signal the presence of toxic metals and other pollutants. If the patient has allergies then they would be expected to reveal their existence during a screening test. Of possibly greater interest to a conventional doctor is that it is possible to identify an overdose, raised cholesterol, high blood pressure, pre-diabetes, raised urea, raised uric acid and low blood levels of oxygen.

Following the screening tests, of which the above represents only a proportion of the available measurements, it is then possible to make a more detailed investigation. The Vega machine enables the operator to assess the function of every single organ in the body. It is even possible to subdivide and to test the various organs of the body. If there are tests missing in the machine for any small anatomical parts of the body it is possible to overcome this problem by the use of separate specific test ampoules that can be placed on the machine.

There are four more sections devoted to various allergies. However I find that most of these problems will disappear once the underlying disease has been identified and treated. There follows tests for toxic metals, which may be of more interest to dentists. The next section enables the operator to confirm the presence of fungi, viruses, bacteria and parasites. The machine is even capable of identifying individual organisms, and once again if any doubt persists there are more comprehensive test ampoules available. It is important to note that parasitic infections are very common causes of many diseases including cancer. Parasites are difficult to identify in pathology laboratories and therefore these infections usually pass unnoticed. Conventional, homeopathic and herbal remedies can successfully treat parasites, once identified.

The next section of tests identifies the various deficiencies. Individual deficiencies of hormones, enzymes, vitamins and minerals can be identified. The latter is perhaps the most important test of all because conventional medicine estimates very few minerals. (In all chronic disease there is always some mineral deficiency. In cancer there is invariably a selenium deficiency. Selenium is seldom, if ever, estimated and therefore cancer patients are deprived this most essential treatment.)

The Vega Expert is also an invaluable tool for dentists. It is possible to identify any dental or associated medical disease. It is possible to identify the individual diseased tooth. The machine can identify which dental materials are compatible. If there are electrical currents flowing between different types of metal fillings then the machine can be used to identify and to correct this problem.

The remainder of the tests are principally of interest to alternative practitioners, because they are designed to identify the most appropriate treatments, their dosage, strength and frequency of use.

Cancer, like all other chronic disease, has an underlying pathological cause and consequent mineral, and possibly vitamin, deficiency. In the hands of a competent operator the Vega Expert can, in less than thirty minutes, identify the presence of a cancer, its cause and the inevitable mineral deficiencies. The patient can then, with confidence, be referred for specialist advice and treatment. It is possible to imagine the changes that could take place within the NHS if GPs and hospital practitioners, would embrace these technologies. Patients with serious disease would gain more rapid access to hospital. Other chronic illnesses could be diagnosed and safely treated in the patient's own surgery. Waiting lists would shrink, doctor workloads diminish and most important of all, patients would get greater satisfaction. In a very short time we could progress from having a third world service to a modern health care system like Germany and many other countries. Less of the nation's wealth would be spent upon propping up a failing health care system, and more money could be spent attaining and maintaining good health and other worthwhile causes. For the individual doctor there could be more job satisfaction and he or she could become the controller and conductor of both conventional and alternative medicine.

(b) The information highway of complementary medicine

David Broom

icon December 2003

Bioelectronic machines such as the Vega and BEST machines scan the body by detecting minute changes in the conductance of the skin over acupuncture points. The most advanced devices are mostly computerised these days and store thousands of test ampoules electronically in a memory bank.

Patients can be tested for food and chemical sensitivity, vitamin and mineral deficiencies, viruses, bacteria and parasites.

Also with specialised tissue matching ampoules it is possible to assess and compare organic functions. For example, if the liver is stressed we can obtain a percentage value on a meter scale to monitor progress of the liver and other organ functions in response to dietary changes and medicines given.

Testing procedure
During a typical session with the computerised Vega Expert the patient holds a metal tube connected by a wire to the system. The practitioner touches one of the patient's acupoints with a handheld electrode, which is also connected to the machine. This enables the practitioner to measure the electrical energy of the acupoint on a meter. Test items are then fed into the circuit and the response to each item is noted. For example – if you have a wheat problem the body will react on this 'subtle energy' level and the meter reading will drop – indicating an aversion to the substance.

The effect of different medicines can also be monitored by the resonance reaction, which occurs in testing. Although this sort of device should not be used alone, instead of traditional blood tests to diagnose specific conditions, it has been shown to be extremely accurate in confirming results and also offering extra information to patients to assist them in their personal choices of treatment.

The value of such testing in skilled hands cannot be overestimated in the treatment of cancers of all kinds. The multi-dimensional nature of chronic disease requires a full understanding of each individual and this has to include knowledge of nutritional balance and how the body is reacting to food, chemicals and medicines. We also need to be aware of the effects of parasites in the body – particularly since these can undermine the health by blocking the proper absorption of essential vitamins and minerals. 'One man's meat is another's poison" is certainly true in the area of nutrition.

Cancer and parasites
Recently an American doctor Hulda Clark has put forward the theory that most chronic disease involves parasite attack in the body, and she believes that we can assist recovery from chronic illness if we are able to identify and destroy these invaders.

For instance – Fasciolopsi buski is a fluke, which she claims she has found present in every case of cancer that she has investigated. Apparently the same fluke is found in sufferers from Alzheimer's disease, Chrohns, Kaposis and Endometriosis. These adult flukes live in the intestine and can produce 1000 eggs per bowel movement and live many years. When the immune system is sound these parasites and others will not survive long enough to cause damage but in the presence of pollutants such as chemical pesticides and particularly isopropyl alcohol, benzene, wood alcohol and toluene – all chemicals found in profusion in the modern world – they thrive and develop to the adult stage.

Yeast is another problem. It seems that most people have too much yeast in their bodies due to prescribed antibiotics and the high levels found in animal feeds. The rapid spread of bugs like MRSA in hospitals tells us that antibiotics are not dealing effectively with new types of bacteria.

Testing a wide range of items can help patients to make necessary corrections to their lifestyles and diets – thus reducing risk factors and strengthening body systems which have become disabled

A common mould known as aflatoxin B is found in large quantities when parasites are present. It is believed that this could create a carcinogenic environment for the host. Since vitamin C has been found to neutralise aflatoxins it would be important to know about any deficiency of this vital vitamin by testing. The need to supplement would be further substantiated if the patient demonstrates the presence of aflatoxin B.

Bioelectronic testing is really the information highway of complementary medicine and will undoubtedly find its way into the mainstream of medicine. Meanwhile the technology is out there and available for you to try. As with any therapy it is wise to seek the counsel of well-established practitioners when dealing with chronic disease conditions.

Communicating with our cells
Scientists working with bioelectronics have suggested that cancer might be a disease in which the normal electron signal, which regulates cell division, has gone wild. Cells emit weak bursts of UV light, which is one of the ways in which they communicate with each other.

Russian scientists made a remarkable discovery 50 years ago when they placed cell

cultures side by side in quartz dishes. When a poison was added to each of the cultures, the cells in both culture dishes died a 'mirror image' death.

This meant that there had to be a transfer of cellular information, which had 'jumped' from one dish to the other. This same effect does not occur if we use glass containers as glass blocks UV light. From this we can deduce that UV light emission is vital to cell communication.

Light to treat cancers
Cancer therapies today are using different frequencies of light to activate the cancer killing properties of certain types of medicine.

Photodynamic Therapy uses light sensitive dyes, which selectively kill cancer cells while leaving the surrounding tissue unharmed. This is being used for basal and squamous cell carcinomas of the skin.

The introduction of 'light' therapies to the current medical agenda for cancer treatments has its counterpart in the growing interest in 'Bioelectrography' in the complementary arena. This is a term used when showing the effects of the body's aura (electrical field) in health and disease.

Kirlian photography
This is the name given to the special techniques of aura photography that were originally developed by Semion Kirlian during the Russian Revolution. Dr Konstantin Korotkov from St Petersburg University is at the forefront of bioelectrography research and development and has invented a device based on this knowledge – called GDV (Gas Discharge Visualisation), which I have found very useful in everyday practice. This equipment is certified by the Russian government for use in clinics and hospitals and shows a magnetic field around the body. All Kirlian photographs are taken within a high frequency energy field and reveal the invisible scaffolding around us known as the human aura.

Within minutes of taking photos of the acupuncture points around the fingers we can construct a whole body image, which shows the level or balance or disturbance in specific areas. From this we can see graphically what is happening energetically within the patient. We are also able to observe the 'aura' in real time on the computer screen as the photograph is being taken.

Using this equipment, we have also been able to demonstrate the energy fields around foods and other substances. This provides information about the quality of food – particularly when grown to organic methods. The Biophotons or light emissions from items tested vary considerably and are much less in poor quality products.

Interestingly we have found that food cooked by microwaves loses its essential quality of biophoton emission and is therefore not recommended. Eating food is considered to be a kind of transference of light energy to the cells of the body. The same principle applies to food grown organically compared to food grown with pesticides and herbicides present in the soil. Organic food has a better biophoton output – more light energy – and in my opinion is therefore better for us.

We are bathed in a sea of light energies and it seems that we are now progressing towards an understanding of 'light' and the more 'subtle energies' as effective agents in the healing process.

Kirlian photographs and cancer
Surveys in Russia demonstrate a significant increase in the ability to diagnose cancers using the GDV device. In randomised blind experiments with 280 patients in Georgia Oncology Center, Marina Shaduri was 85–95 per cent correct in her evaluation of different kinds of cancer.

This same researcher was able to make a detailed analysis of different parts of the digestive tract, individual sections of the head and organs – including the measurement of the level of urine in the bladder.

Harry Oldfield, a British pioneer in this field, discovered that if you probe the area over a tumour with a kind of Kirlian gun, the frequency and polarity characteristics of the signal would become distorted. A pilot study of cancer patients at Charing Cross Hospital showed accuracy in pinpointing the specific location of tumours. Oldfield used several probes at different angles around the body and found that he could mathematically triangulate to calculate the tumour's depth and the exact location of the tumour.

Professor Korotkov, inventor of the GDV device, is using the photos of blood plasma to detect changes relevant to cancer diagnostics.

In general practice
To summarise: the use of Bioelectronic Testing and Kirlian Photography and its modern equivalent, the GDV device, can help in the following ways:

1 We can observe the interactions between diseased and stressed organs and the whole body.
2 Patients can be monitored during treatments so that a more effective valuation of that treatment can be made.
3 Pathological processes can be observed through the images present (further research will undoubtedly provide a dictionary of information).
4   We can observe healing processes taking place.

These Bioelectronic systems in skilled hands can provide patients with information vital to their recovery. The use of what is described as 'subtle energy techniques' can lead us onto even greater discoveries about how the body works which in turn will help us all to gain the knowledge necessary to defeat suffering and disease.

21 Zap that cancer

Ginny Fraser

icon February 2004

Anyone taking charge of dealing with their cancer will have extensively explored the medical treatments available. They will have read widely about diet, and made significant changes. They will probably have stopped using toxic substances – from cigarettes and sugar to certain brands of bathroom cleaner. They will be exercising and taking supplements. It will feel like no stone has been left unturned.

There is, however, a little-known area that may provide another weapon in the cancer patient's arsenal – *electronic medicine.*

The claims made about this technology are dramatic, with some of its proponents claiming you can literally zap your cancer into submission in the comfort of your own home, using a device called – and here is the technical term – a zapper!

Parasites as the cause
Best-known proponent of the zapper is American researcher, Hulda Clark, author of the confidently titled *The Cure for All Cancers*. The basic principle behind her work is that ALL cancers are caused by a combination of two factors – first that everyone with cancer has parasites, particularly intestinal, liver and pancreatic flukes and the common roundworm. The second factor is the presence of solvents in the body (through pollution of the food chain). Different solvents accumulate preferentially in different organs, giving rise to different diseases. Isopropyl alcohol, for instance, accumulates in the liver. According to Clark, this results in the completion of the life cycle of the fluke

(fasciolopsis buskii) in the liver, which establishes the malignant process.

Clark claims that the removal of solvents from the patient's body and environment plus the killing of the parasites and their larvae results in a "remarkable recovery". The zapper is part of her regime to do this, as is an extremely stringent detoxification regime that is almost impossible for anyone not living on top of a mountain in New Zealand, and includes things like getting rid of pets and removal of fillings and sometimes teeth.

The principle behind Clark's zapper is resonance. This is what happens when an opera singer hits a high note and a glass shatters. The same thing happens when you rub a finger around the top of a wine glass and it resonates. Just like the glass, all bacteria and pathogens have a frequency. Clark's research claims "Any positive offset (DC) frequency kills all bacteria, viruses and parasites simultaneously given sufficient voltage (five to 10 volts), duration (seven minutes) and frequency (anything from 10 Hz to 500,000 Hz). A treatment cycle of three blocks of seven minutes, separated by 20-minute gaps is recommended. Clark recommends that users zap daily for two to three weeks and then once weekly thereafter. It is completely painless and most people don't really feel much, although some report a slight warming of the hands.

There has been no rigorous research done on the Clark approach and all the evidence is anecdotal. She claims to have 'cured' 100 people of cancer with her methods before she went public with her theory, and over the past fifteen years has treated over 2,000 patients. She is currently facing prosecution by the Federal Trade Commission in the US over 'unsubstantiated representations' made about her products and devices including the zapper.

So the jury is still out on the efficiency of the Clark zapper. However, for anyone wanting to experiment, it is relatively cheap and can be self-assembled even more cheaply from the instructions in her book. We doubt it can do harm, provided her instructions are followed.

Electrical zapping
Less well-known is the Beck zapper. The principle behind it was discovered at the Albert Einstein College of Medicine in New York in 1991. Researchers found that when the HIV virus was exposed to a small current it lost its ability to infect white blood cells. The current damages the outside of the micro-organisms making them weaker and more vulnerable to attack by the body's natural defence system. This is a different fundamental principle to the Clark machine.

The electrodes of the Beck zapper are placed on the ankles, and the sensation feels like an electrical thump alternately at each ankle. The amount of power going into each electrode can be adjusted to suit you, and treatment sessions are usually around an hour. It is recommended that you build up the usage by 15 minutes a week for three weeks until you reach one hour. Use the zapper then for another week at one hour per day; rest for one week, then zap every three weeks with the fourth week off. The reason for the cautious approach is not that the zapper itself will cause any damage, but to avoid the toxic overload that the zapped matter can cause to the liver and kidneys. Two and a half litres of water per day are recommended to assist in the flushing of the toxins.

Beck makes very cautious claims about what his device can help with. He calls it simply a blood purifier, but theoretically it can be beneficial in cancer, HIV and any other systemic invaders in the blood. Unlike other machines, however, it only works on the blood.

In the UK, Chris Hyslop of Commercial Science is enthusiastic about the Beck machine, and sells both it and the Clark models. Formerly a microbiologist, Hyslop now works as a homeopath and thus has a keen interest in healing generally. His personal experience with the Beck machine is compelling. After a fourteen-day bout of serious flu, he had weeks of post-viral fatigue syndrome that was proving impossible to shift. Being involved in complementary therapies he tried fourteen different treatments to no avail. A friend lent him the Beck machine, and overnight he had a huge improvement. "I felt like I'd been switched back on," he says. Tests done by Hyslop with the Beck machine showed that it "significantly slowed down growth rates of bacteria, yeasts and moulds in the test tube compared with non-treated controls". Commercial Science's research with the Clark zapper did not appear to have any effect, though the tests were done *in vitro* and Hyslop acknowledges that *in vivo* results might be very different. It is recommended that for cancer, the Beck zapper, which costs under a hundred pounds to purchase, be used in conjunction with colloidal silver, magnetic pulsing and ozonated water.

Royal Rife
In another league altogether are the machines based around the technology of Dr Royal Rife. The story of Rife and his incredible scientific discoveries is one surrounded by intrigue.

Working in the USA in 1931, Rife came to the attention of the scientific world with a microscope of extraordinary magnification and resolution. His breakthrough was well-documented in the most prestigious scientific journals. In 1932, using his powerful microscope, he saw a virus at the heart of every solid tumour (which he called BX), and at the heart of every diffuse cancer (BY). He then identified a radio frequency that destroyed only the virus while he watched. Decades later this accomplishment remained unrivalled, and the supporters of Rife claim that there has been nothing to touch his discoveries to this day. His success with cancer patients lay in the fact that his powerful microscope allowed him to work out very precisely which frequencies killed the microbes without damaging anything else.

By the mid-thirties work was in progress at the University of Southern California to bring Rife's discoveries to the world. At the same time the American Medical Association had a strong focus of opposition to 'energy medicine', and was purportedly run by those who had close connections with the pharmaceutical industry. A series of investigations into Rife and his technologies began and the story goes that the laboratory in New Jersey where his investigations were being checked was burned down. The full story of Dr Rife can be found in Barry Lynes book *The Cancer Cure that Worked*. According to Lynes, writing in the California Sun, "The world was on the verge of a medical-scientific revolution that, if it had taken place, would have brought a totally different kind of health practice and science to the human family."

The story continues with the mysterious disappearance of records and Rife's technologies were basically lost to the world. He died in 1971 a broken man.

However, today there are a number of people trying to re-create what Rife discovered, and Rife-inspired machines are available. One of the most respected of these is the Rife-Bare machine developed by James Bare. This has been approved by Health Canada (the equivalent of the USA's FDA), but remains outlawed in the USA.

The Rife-Bare machine uses a gas plasma tube to radiate energy to the patient. It looks a bit like a vertical neon light tube. The patient must be between six to twelve feet away from the machine, and can quite happily do other activities while being 'zapped'. Bare makes no claims for curing cancer, and there is no quality research on its effectiveness, but he cites plenty of anecdotal evidence where it has been effective with cancer. Rife's original machine was used with a 100 per cent success rate on trials with 16 patients with advanced cancer. The Rife-Bare machine has also shown promising results. A volunteer-based evaluation programme has been running since 1996, and volunteers have reported "reduction in the size of tumours, reduction of pain and inflammation". Again, not very scientific, but all the results are viewable at www.resonantlight.com.

In England it is necessary to import a machine from Canada at a cost of around £2000, or make one yourself, based on James Bare's detailed instructions (see his book *Resonant Frequency Therapy: Building the Rife/Bare Beam Ray Device*, available through www.rt66.com).

The field of electronic frequency medicine is not new, but it is still unproven. For those who want to explore all the options it certainly deserves a deeper investigation. As with any treatment – conventional and alternative – check it out. The Internet allows us unprecedented access to information. An **icon** volunteer has also conducted an experiment with a Rife-Bare machine on a user with melanoma. Results will be measured by CT scan, and we will have to include them in the second edition of this book! Sorry!

Clark and Beck zappers are available from Commercial Science on www.comsci.org.uk.

22 A virus at the heart of every cancer?

The work of Dr Royal Rife
by Chris Woollams

First some elementary biology: Viruses are a unique group of organisms. They grow inside other cells, for example those of bacteria, fungi, plants or animals. They do not have a full cellular structure, like an animal cell, of nucleus, power station, cell membranes or of a central DNA strand sending out messenger RNA to convey demands to the cell and the organism outside. They are very basic with a protein shell surrounding the vital genetic code (which may be DNA or RNA). In order to replicate they must take control of a host cell and order its DNA to produce proteins and all that is necessary for the multiplication of the virus.

In fact, the virus genetic code over-rides and misdirects the cell's own genetic code.

So that will be very similar to what happens in a cancer cell then! Indeed, in both cases the host cell's DNA loses its 'normal' production control.

'Viruses' like, for example, radiation or toxic chemicals can mutate the master control DNA and cause rogue cell production and cancer too.

The National Cancer Institute in the USA lists the following as 'some viruses associated with human cancers'.

Epstein-Barr	Burkitt's Lymphoma
Human papillomavirus	Cervical cancer

Hepatitis B virus	Liver cancer
Human T-cell lymphatic virus	T-cell leukaemia
Kaposi's sarcoma virus	Kaposi's sarcoma!

They also confirm that Helicobacter pylori, a bacteria which can cause stomach ulcers has been associated with the development of stomach cancers.

To this list can be added the following microbes and possible links.

HTLV-1	(a type of Japanese Leukaemia)
Hepatitis C	Liver cancer
Retro-virus (HTLV-2)	Hairy-cell leukaemia
Grannloma type virus	Skin cancer

One mystery of the possibility that viruses cause cancer is that, for example, 90 per cent of British adults have Epstein Barr virus but most come to no harm, even though it is now linked not just to Burkitt's lymphoma but Hodgkin's disease, nasopharynual cancer and a few rarer cancers. It does seem that it can inactivate a gene (*p16*), which is a normal cell defender (*Journal of Cell Biology*).

Overall, Cancer Research UK feels that 15–20 per cent of all cancers may have viral cause, but new discoveries are being made all the time.

In April 2004 scientists at the University of Pittsburgh found that 20 to 40 per cent of men with prostate cancer carried the cold sore virus, a herpes variant, in their bloodstream. That is twice the level of those with no cancer. It is already know that another variant of the herpes virus is causal in cervical cancer.

However, since the vast majority of adults carry the herpes virus, the crucial question is 'What is turning it on in some cases and not other?' Scientists monitored women with cervical cancer and found they lacked human leukocyte antigen (HLA).

The majority of women who were able to overcome any herpes infection had HLA present in their abnormal cells.

But the question remains how does this virus cause the cancer, if at all. It could simply be that it so weakens the immune system, the host is more vulnerable.

The whole virus/cancer issue has come more and more to the fore over the last five or so years largely led by the PR departments of some pharmaceutical companies that have developed vaccines. For example, Merck have developed a vaccine that can prevent women being affected by two forms of Human papillomavirus (HPV), which account for 70 per cent of cervical cancers. Since HPV is sexually transmitted, the long-term idea presumably is that all girls could be vaccinated before their first sexual encounter. That sounds like big business!

It was not always thus. In the 1960s and 1970s, US virologists put a lot of effort into studying possible viral causes of cancer, and their impact on tumour suppressor genes like *p53*, *ras* and *myc*. However, the technology was not particularly on their side and little was found. This coupled with euphoria about drugs and chemotherapy put the work on the back burner.

By the mid-1990s however knowledge and technology had improved dramatically and coupled with the prospect of more profitable vaccines across populations as a whole, viral studies have become trendy again. New work is breaking out everywhere.

In a paper from Tulane University (February 2004), avian viruses have become prime suspects for some human cancers. Eric Johnson, associate professor of epidemiology studied poultry workers in Baltimore and Missouri. Chicken viruses are killed when the chicken is cooked, but can you 'catch' it from raw meat? The Baltimore study showed that the poultry workers had four times the expected rate of oesophageal cancer, while workers in Missouri had higher rates of lung, kidney, pancreas, blood or lymphatic cancers.

Two types of retrovirus exist in chickens – avian leukaemia and sarcoma virus; and reiculoendotheliosis virus (REV). Each can kill a chicken within a week of infection. What if these viruses could pass to humans? They can infect human cells in laboratory tests, so now Johnson is looking for them in the DNA of humans.

And then there are mice.

Another retrovirus is the mouse mammary tumour virus (MMTV). Discovered in 1930 it causes breast cancer, albeit in mice. The 'virus hypothesis' of a link from mice to women came about through epidemiology studies. Thomas Steward of the University of Ottawa learned that human breast cancer incidence coincides with the habitat of *mus domesticus*, the mouse species with MMTV. Both were most prevalent in the USA and Western Europe, and the suggested link was through fleas, anthropods or mosquitoes (*BJC* January 2000).

However, all early work failed to find any connection or transmission in the laboratory. A theory that just a sequence of the virus is linked to breast cancer is also in debate, and there are also claims that viral proteins have been found in breast tissue (Beatrice Pogo, Mount Sinai School of Medicine).

The American jury is currently undecided.

However scientists at the University of New South Wales have been looking into the possibility of a breast cancer virus for some time and they found in 2000 that 42 per cent of breast cancer patients tested did indeed have the virus compared to only 2 per cent of healthy breasts. Their research in 2002 showed the virus was only located in the tumours and not in the surrounding healthy tissue.

By 2003 in the *Clinical Cancer Research Journal*, they had reported that the virus was found in Australian women but not Vietnamese. Caroline Ford from the University argued that women were often told that breast cancer was in some way hereditary. But the fact was that genetics only accounted for 5–6 per cent of possible cause leaving 95 per cent unexplained.

Of course, if a viral connection can be proven, there will be a rush to develop a vaccine. For all women – although an alternative might be to sort out the mice, I suppose!

Already Dr Robert Garry of Tulane is noting that certain vertebrate species other than mice have a mammary virus. Dr Orli Etingin, Assistant Professor at Cornell Medical Centre, New York, says this is all very interesting. Retroviruses have been implicated in lymphomas and it is possible they do link to tumours in humans.

The truth may be that the issue is not as simple as a virus in one host becoming a virus in another. A discovery was made in 1975 was that some viruses in animals were RNA viruses i.e. not DNA viruses but more like the messages sent out by human DNA within the cell. Dr Robert Simpson of Rutgears University found that some RNA viruses could infect human cells and form a DNA pro-virus, harmless and dormant for long periods. Some examples he gave were influenza, measles, mumps and polio viruses.

Certainly in the 1960s there was panic in US medical circles over the Salk polio vaccine. Salk mass-produced the vaccine by growing it on the kidneys of rhesus monkeys. However, after five or so years of its use, researchers identified that there was a viral contaminate, SV-40, from the monkeys. When this was injected into animals it produced brain tumours. By 1963 the rhesus monkey had been replaced by the African green monkey but in the preceding eight years, 98 million Americans had been vaccinated!

SV-40 appears in 61 per cent of all new cancer patients; patients often too young to have received the vaccine. Dr Howard Strickler at the US National Institute of Health has plotted a geographic profile linking the SV-40 to the tainted vaccine. And the findings are very worrying. For example, people who lived in Massachusetts and Illinois and who received the contaminated vaccine now have more than 10 times the rate of bone tumours. And the fear is that this pro-virus can now pass human to human.

Now researchers in Japan (*Cancer Research* 2003 63, 7606) warn that SV-40 may be spreading throughout the human population leaving cancer in its wake. It is now known to be linked to a number of cancers including malignant mesothelioma, various brain tumours and non-Hodgkins lymphoma. SV-40 is known to produce large T-antigens that block your cellular protector genes like *p53*. The Japanese researchers found SV-40 present in up to 19 per cent of some cancer cases, none of which had been exposed to Salk polio vaccine.

But what if something unknown to date could then turn a provirus on?

What if, not 15 per cent, but all cancers were in some way linked to viruses or viral elements as catalysts or cause?

Genes and cancer
In every cell of your body you have a nucleus, and within that lies your DNA, your master code; the blueprint for your whole body.

Along that string of DNA lie thousands of genes, each a little message for the colour of your eyes or the size of your nose.

Three groups of these genes are important in cancer.

1. Proto-oncogenes
Proteins called 'growth factors' normally control cell growth and division and the controlling genes for these are proto-oncogens.

These bind to receptors on the cell membrane and tell the inside of the cell to make a copy of itself. Sometimes the proto-oncogens have gone 'wrong', causing odd growth factors to be found, which in turn tell the cell to do 'odd things'. These 'wrong' genes (formed because somehow the proto-oncogens have been damaged), are called oncogenes.

These oncogenes act like petrol on the receptor sites causing the whole cell to start dividing madly.

2. Tumour suppressor genes
Inside the DNA string we normally have defender genes. One example is called p53. Its job is to spot when the DNA system has gone wrong and cause the self-destruction of the cell. There are a number of these genes, but sometimes they themselves go wrong leaving the cell unprotected.

3. DNA repair genes
Also contained in your normal DNA string are a number of genes whose job it is to 'spot' imperfections in, for example, the copying process and tell the DNA to repair itself. Again sometimes these genes go wrong leaving the cell without its in-store repairmen.

BRCA1 and BRCA2 were originally identified as genes that went wrong in breast cancer. They afflict about 6 per cent of women. However it is now known that they afflict men too and are in fact not breast cancer genes but tumour suppressor and repair genes.

Dr Royal Raymond Rife

Back in the early 1930s the idea that there was a virus at the heart of every tumour is exactly what Dr Rife thought.

Unfortunately the story that surrounds this man's life's work is nothing short of scandalous.

Royal Raymond Rife, a scientist, started working in San Diego in 1915 and from 1920 invented a totally new kind of microscope. Such was the magnification he claimed, that it would be 10 times more powerful than even today's best microscopes. It was an amazing advance as also, unlike existing electron microscopes, Rife's microscope could view **living** bacteria and viruses.

His work covered all manner of illnesses but it was with cancer he achieved his notoriety.

Using his microscope to study tumours, Rife claimed he could see a cancer-causing substance inside the tumour. This factor he identified as bacterial, but he then argued that with his microscope he could see it change shape and form, and even develop viral properties.

The shape change and indeed the cancer-causing factor's release depended upon the medium in which it lived. He claimed quite simply that in certain conditions the cancer factor was inert or neutral, whilst in others it became active.

Instead of working on these medium changes, he started beaming light at the microorganism but he claimed to be able to find a frequency to each, so that he could both see and also by using electrical currents, 'blow up' microorganisms involved in a variety of illnesses like TB, leprosy, anthrax, herpes, cancer and many more.

Over the forty years from 1920 to 1960 he conducted extensive research. He obtained his pathogenic organisms from top medical clinics like the Mayo Clinic, he had one of the best privately equipped laboratories in the world and his own high powered microscopes he designed and built for the isolation of cancer and other 'viruses'. His microscope was fully described in a publication called the *Journal of the Franklin Institute*.

In fact, he claimed to have isolated forty or more viruses never isolated before including 'cancer virus' which he obtained from breast cells. In each case he 'saw' them by shining light of a particular frequency on them through his 'prismatic virus microscope'.

A number of doctors and other scientists worked with him during his studies, not just in San Diego but also all over the USA. As part of his studies, Rife even took his cancer-causing factors and implanted them into rats. Cancer tumours formed.

Obviously though the big step was to study cancers actually in humans, rather than under microscopes. The medical research committee of the University of Southern California and Doctor Milbank Johnson, MD oversaw the first clinical study. Sixteen people, each with different cancers in terminal forms were treated and fourteen were clear within three months. Dr Alvin G Feord, a clinical pathologist, confirmed this. In 1939 Rife addressed the Royal Society of Medicine in London and they approved his findings.

In the late 1930s and 1940s Rife's work was being developed in other parts of America notably by Dr Stafford in Ohio and Dr James Couche. Milbank Johnson, a millionaire, funded three clinics, working in one himself for 8 years. Dr Arthur Kendall, Director of Medical Research at North Western University and Rife published a full report of their studies in the *Journal of the Californian Medical Association*, and Dr Rosenow of the Mayo Clinic observed other studies, which he in turn published.

Work now needed to change gear. If live human beings were to be treated a methodology for delivering the correct resonance frequency into the tumours had to be perfected. During the 1950s Rife worked with his engineer John Crane to build an improved type of 'frequency device', using electrodes, which could be placed on the body to provide the resonance waves to kill the virus. Together they formed the Rife Ray Beam Tube Corporation.

By 1960, some 90 resonance machines had been built and distributed for use across America, and even in England.

Various scientists and doctors used them all claiming great successes.

But life was starting to go wrong.

Although Rife and others had asked the Department of Health, The American Cancer Society, The Sloan-Kettering Institute and many others to review their work, all declined. The American Cancer Society did show some interest until they found out that neither Rife nor Crane were medical doctors. No one seemed interested in an electronic frequency as a method of curing cancer.

Rife requested that medical schools reviewed his work and this did take place at the Hooper Foundation of the University of California and at Northwestern Medical School but still no Medical Authority was interested.

In 1960 the American Medical Association apparently raided Crane's laboratories without a search warrant and what they didn't remove, they smashed. Crane was taken to trial in 1961 by which time Rife was 72 and living out of reach of the authorities in Mexico. At Crane's trial no evidence was allowed from any doctor, or any research trial, and Crane was jailed for illegally treating patients. 14 patients did testify, but the prosecution instead used the opinion of Dr Paul Shea, who had been given a frequency machine two months before and had never even turned it on. Yet, Dr Shea testified that it could have no curative powers. The foreman of the jury was apparently an AMA doctor, and Crane was sentenced to ten years in jail, which following appeal was cut. He served three years.

Various other practitioners like Dr Stafford in Ohio gave up their studies and the work finished.

Of course, the really sad thing is that all this happened over 50 years ago. How much more could have been learned if work had continued? About the same time the Russians actually started their research on body energy and noted that each organ has its own particular frequency, as indeed does a cancer cell. The Russians continue their work on resonance machines; one such machine is the Oberon machine and the Dove Clinic in the UK has an example.

Whether there are viruses or bacterial factors at the heart of all cancers is a question that still hasn't actually been answered, 75 years after Rife invented his microscope. How crazy is that?

And whilst placing electrodes on people around their tumours may have been a crude way of treating them with a resonance frequency that might kill cancer cells, the principle is undoubtedly correct. MRI scans use the principle of differing frequencies of organs and cancer cells every day of the week in oncology units.

Rife died in 1971, a broken man. If more and more cancers are found to have a viral cause, and Rife's experiments can be replicated and advanced we may yet have a cure for cancer, one that can be purchased and used in every home. And maybe Dr Royal Rife will be afforded the place in history he deserves.

But arguably the saddest part to all this, and one that feeds the conspiracy theorists, is simply that the work was just dismissed. Not reviewed, not developed, not logically and scientifically appraised, just dismissed.

Barry Lynes, a journalist, wrote a book called *The Cancer Cure that Worked! 50 Years of Suppression*. Now at least some scientists have been finding examples, in Germany and the UK, of the Rife-Crane machines and we may yet see some commonsense prevail with new studies and scientific tests conducted under the auspices of the authorities. Especially as more and more studies seem to find viruses and other such factors at the root of cancers.

23 Using viruses to treat cancer

Chris Woollams

Virotherapy is a fast emerging 'treatment of potential' in cancer therapies. Read this article from Cancer Watch in **icon** magazine to understand it a little more:

MD Anderson celebrates gene therapy success
Back in 1997, Dr Jack Roth of the MD Anderson Cancer Centre pioneered work using a genetically engineered virus, with human lung cancer patients. Five years on they are celebrating the results. Two patients (Alfredo Gonzalvo, now 78 and Bernis Teaters, now 84) became medical pioneers by having the treatment in conjunction with 6 weeks of radiotherapy. Roth used an adenovirus (the bug that causes the common cold) as a vector to take in healthy copies of the p53 gene, right into the lung cancer tumours. The therapy is currently on fast track FDA approval

The pioneering work started with a premise: The p53 gene, which normally acts to suppress uncontrolled cell growth, is missing or mutated in about 50 per cent of human cancers, and dysfunctional in the rest. So let's get the p 53 gene back inside the tumour to regulate the cancer growth and normalise the cells.

The therapy, called Advexin, has shrunk lung tumours in over half the patients trialled. Both the above named patients were treated in May 1999, and are celebrating their fifth anniversary.

MD Anderson has run more than 20 trials to date, featuring 600 patients. Advexin has been used in lung, head and neck, breast *and ovarian tumours, whilst other viruses have been tested with brain tumours and metastatic lung cancers.*

The only hiccough to date has been a tendency for immune response in patients, but Roth is now using genes encased in liposomes which act like shrink-wrapping to get the active ingredient past the healthy cells and into the tumour.

The principle is simple. First find your virus, and then train it to specifically attack tumour cells. This 'training' usually involves gene modification so that healthy cells can recognise it and destroy it leaving it only a problem for the cancer cells. There it could cause lysis and destroy the tumour, it could deliver therapeutic genes, or even specific anti-cancer drugs.

Such self-replicating viruses have already been tested both in vitro and in vivo. They can be used instead of radio and chemotherapy, or alongside it without affecting healthy cells.

Example 1: Daniel Meruelo (New York University School of Medicine) has undertaken pre-clinical trials and shown that Sindbis virus can target ovarian, kidney, stomach, colon and advanced pancreatic cancers (*Nat Biotechnol* 2004, 22: 70-77). To date Meruelo has done his tests with mice, but given the poor progress with pancreatic and ovarian cancers he hopes to begin human trials within 2–3 years.

Example 2: Darren Shafren (University of Newcastle NSW) showed that coxsackievirus A21 causes lysis and complete destruction of melanomas. He has undertaken this research in vitro and in mice. The CVA21 virus is an enterovirus; it causes the common cold. Just one injected dose directed into the tumours caused their destruction. The melanoma actually seems to cause rapid multiplication of the virus.

Work is taking place in the UK too. Again read this short piece from **icon**:

UK gene therapy trial for brain tumours
Notwithstanding the MD Anderson work, Professor Norman Nevin, chair of the UK gene therapy committee believes the UK is at the forefront of their type of work. His committee has given the go-ahead for a team at Glasgow University, lead by Professor Moira Brown, to treat 100 patients with gliomas using a genetically modified form of the herpes virus.

In the normal brain, this virus can cause encephalitis. But this modified virus has a gene removed so that it leaves normal cells unharmed but replicates in a cancer cell, causing them to burst open, and spread the disease to other cancer cells.

39 patients have been involved in three previous trials. Currently orthodox medicine has no cure for gliomas. But one is still alive from a 1997 trial and five from a more recent trial. All greatly exceeded their doctor's diagnosis, as did a number of other patients in the trial. Brown added that this was the most advanced gene therapy trial in the UK.

There are a number of implications and questions that still need answers.

In the melanoma study, the virus multiplied and headed off around the body to other, distant tumours. All this on a very low initial viral dose. Where does the virus stop?

The mice used in the experiments all had immune deficiency – so that they didn't kick out the virus. How will that translate into human therapy? Already the M D Anderson team are acknowledging that immune response is a problem and so they are coating – and thus hiding – their virus from healthy cells.

Will it work for late stage disease as well as it does for early stage? To what degree is the immune deficiency essential? And what are the side effects and risks?

So, early days yet, but researchers all over the world are

working in this field using viruses like adenovirus, herpesvirus (on breast cancers) and poliovirus.

24 Recharging your failing cells

The work of Dr David Walker
Chris Woollams

A biophysicist's approach to curing colon cancer
In 1994 David Walker, a 40-year-old Doctor of Biophysics, had an appendix operation, and discovered he had colon cancer with metastasis to five other organ locations. He undertook a course of chemotherapy and followed his oncologist's orders.

Unfortunately the surgery left his left leg unusable for six months, whilst the chemotherapy took the skin off the palms of his hands, and generally so poisoned him that he was advised to stop for a period of 3 months. Dr Walker never returned for further chemotherapy treatment.

This was the moment that changed his life. Dr Walker isn't 'just' a Doctor of Biophysics, he has qualifications in both biochemistry and microbiology and set out to do his homework, searching the Internet, reading books and delving in-depth into nutrition, the biochemistry of cancer and its biophysical properties. And then he started his own programme. He detoxed, he took glycoproteins and phytonutrients, and he cut red meat and sugar. All sensible steps and those found every month in **icon**. But his additional and crucial element was unusual, and way outside the knowledge of his doctors.

Cancer cells are low in energy
Just as your body is surrounded by an energetic aura, so is each one of your cells. Made of energetic atoms, and producing energy in the mitochondria or power stations, every healthy cell has a natural energy of between 70 and 90 millivolts.

However not all cells are this 'energised'. For example, free radicals can rip pieces off healthy cell membranes causing them to lose charge down to about 15 millivolts. Dr Walker found that cells with reduced energy levels cannot complete the normal cellular cycle and are more likely to mutate.

Under normal conditions the *p53* gene in all of us destroys mutated cells. It is the 'protector' gene and the 'repairer'. However it needs a certain energy level to do this and 15 millivolts simply is not enough. Thus the *p53* gene, now classified as 'Wild Type *p53*', is rendered inactive – its 'battery' just can't provide enough energy to light the light.

However, Dr Walker then found that another gene (the *myg* gene), which causes cells to divide, could work at levels below 15 millivolts. Being the last gene in the life cycle of communication, known as a life sustention gene, the *myg* gene needs very little energy to do its work. In a mutated cell configuration, this necessary gene then becomes the bad gene, dividing at an accelerated rate causing cancer to grow faster. This stage of damage now results in DNA fragmentation and RNA supplementation, rendering the cell helpless to recognise its own proper structure and means of healthy cellular communication.

So free radicals damage cells and create the activation and acceleration process of the *myg* gene, which, instead of protecting healthy cells, produces mutations; and simultaneously the *p53* protective gene is shut down. Result: cancer.

A multitude of cancer factors
He also researched many of the other factors we frequently mention in **icon**. That cancer cells cannot live in an oxygen-rich environment and that the high levels of oxygen can kill them; that high potassium and magnesium are good for cells and sodium is bad; that glycoproteins help cells communicate and the immune system to 'detect' rogue cells.

In all he identified a number of unique factors in the cycle of cellular communication that had failed in the cancer process and needed to be regenerated to return the cellular systems to health. And thus he developed his own 'therapy'.

Dr Walker's treatment therapy programme

Detoxification: As with Gerson, Plaskett and Gonzalez, detoxification of the blood system and liver was a crucial start point.

Nutrition: He avoided red meat, sugar, hydrogenated vegetable oils, refined carbohydrates and dairy.

He added phytonutrients (e.g. kelp, spirulina) and glycoproteins into his diet.

He supplemented with a variety of anti-cancer supplements and also strongly recommends a herbal enzyme supplement called Bio-X, aka CNX formula, which contains herbs like liquorice root.

Oxygen: At **icon** we encourage people to oxygenate their cells through exercise. Dr Walker used sodium micelle, an enzyme, to do the job.

Bioresonance: David Broom referred to this in his chapter. There are a number of machines on the market that resonate across a spectrum of frequencies. Your different cells and organs each have their own frequency and can pick up on the appropriate signal provided by a resonance machine and thus recharge themselves. The Russians have used similar machines for years in their space programme.

The mission

As Dr Walker treated himself, he became well to the point where after two years his doctor had pronounced him clear of colon, or indeed any, cancer.

Word gets around and people with cancer contacted him. In many instances he helped people with his time and products for free. He even kept detailed records on every patient – over 500 in all, and now after 10 years, he has over 3,500 three-way medical testimonials on his programme and on the products he recommends.

He even asked the National Institute of Health if they would check out his findings. They refused and shortly afterwards the Federal Trade Commission and the Attorney General in association with the FDA sued him on the grounds that, through his website, he was actually providing medical advice. As with Dr Burzynski, the FDA spread its net and over 320 charges were filed against him in three different court cases, from 'selling' illegal over-the-counter drugs to practicing medicine whilst unlicensed.

In the end the Federal Trade Commission decided that it was his 'constitutional right' to review cancer patients' medical records and offer medical advice, but only as long as he didn't sell anything.

Hounded out
Eventually he lost on just two minor charges concerning record keeping and was fined $860,000. This cost him everything he owned, including his home.

Undaunted, he was determined to continue. Although he was offered several jobs in complementary health, he felt he had a mission to accomplish. He knew that existing chemotherapy was damaging and dangerous, whilst he had developed a logical and scientifically justifiable non-toxic alternative. One that delivered results and he had the records to prove it!

So Dr David Walker packed in his life in the USA and set up a clinic in Mexico, where he now consults and designs personalised therapy programmes for cancer and chronic disease patients. Although the days of free service and products are gone, as a result of his poverty due to the US government's actions, the one nice part of his relocation is that one does not have to go to Mexico to get the benefit of this programme, although it is recommended. He has a booklet and can give advice by Internet or phone. This really is not a case of an expensive alternative treatment, nor indeed one that has to be delivered in Mexico for fear of US reprisals.

David is on an honest mission. Often he charges nothing, he just wants to pass on knowledge and help. Interestingly, I was told recently that the Russians have been looking in depth into Bio-resonance, so soon he may not be 'alone' in his theories.

25 Living in harmony

Melanie Hart

icon March/April 2004

If you have a railway line at the bottom of your garden, an electricity substation next door, or pylons and phone masts dotted around your neighbourhood, read on to find out how you can minimise the effects of EMFs (Electric and Magnetic Fields) on your health – other than moving home, of course.

Whatever age we are, whether we're married, single, parents, career-minded or unemployed there's one thing we are all affected by every day – and that's stress. Now, not all stress is toxic. Some is necessary and can be positive, driving us on to achieve things we never thought possible, but, increasingly, the influences of environmental stress are encroaching on our waking and, more importantly, our sleeping hours.

There have been huge transformations in our physical environment in the last few centuries. Housing and transport development has disturbed the natural landscape, and the explosion in communications technology has introduced electro-magnetic fields that permeate our bodies. Some people, including dowsers and kinesiologists Jacqui Beacon and David Gillett, from Environmental Harmony, say that these changes have destroyed the balance of natural forces in the home and workplace, causing three main categories of environmental stress:

Geopathic, caused by distortions in the earth's structure, such as land development and natural movement.

Electro-magnetic, which comes from power-induced electrical appliances and installations. It covers a vast electro-magnetic spectrum, including frequencies used for radar, radio and microwave.

Geopsychic, which is caused by negative thought patterns. These set up resonances, affecting both buildings and land, which may persist for hundreds of years unless cleared.

Researchers around the world have shown that these environmental stresses can trigger or aggravate health problems such as cancer, MS, ME, learning difficulties, allergies, headaches, depression and insomnia. Professor Denis Henshaw of Bristol University has spent years studying the effects of EMFs and has linked them to an increased risk of childhood **leukaemia, brain and other cancers**. As early as 1929, Von Pohl found a connection between geopathic stress and cancer. He dowsed every home in a German village, without knowing anything about the present or previous occupants, and his investigations showed that all the cancer cases and cancer-related deaths in the village had occurred in houses where the underground current was particularly strong (i.e. geopathically stressed).

He advised residents to move their beds, but that is not always possible in today's homes, where space is at a premium. And that's where people like Jacqui and David come in with their home harmonisation skills and range of seven products, including Energy Mixing Beacons. "We balance the whole home so the bed can stay where it is," Jacqui explains. "We can place Energy Mixing Beacons in strategic positions to balance the property, and give the occupants a greater sense of wellbeing. Getting good sleep is very important. EMFs can stop your body repairing itself properly, while you're sleeping, which affects your immune system and leads to illness. People don't realise that it's not just what's in the room that affects you, but what's on the other side of the wall."

One of Jacqui's most memorable visits was to a woman who greeted her on the doorstep saying her goldfish had just died.

And it wasn't the first to have passed away in that house. Jacqui looked around and found a microwave cooker in the kitchen on the other side of the wall. "Every time she turned it on, she was zapping her poor goldfish," Jacqui explains. "All the EMFs were going through the wall and into the goldfish bowl. People don't realise. Some people in flats have the headboards of their beds positioned so that the computer, fridge or cooker is on the other side of the wall. You can imagine what that does for your health!"

Environmental Harmony can work "remotely", by asking a series of questions about the property's location and who lives there, before consulting special maps and 'tuning in' to the property. Jacqui and David then advise on what needs to be done and where to put appropriate products. On-site visits are necessary for complex cases, or when people have serious illnesses. Then the couple use dowsing rods and meters to measure the exact locations and level of the various stresses. They spend around five hours in each property.

"We went to see one lady whose son had epilepsy," Jacqui recalls. "Dave put the Tri-field meter (which measures EMFs) in the bath and it read quite low. Then suddenly it shot right up. All she'd done was turn on the hot tap in the kitchen. We had the same result with the hot taps in the bathroom, which showed us that as soon as the boiler switched on it created a huge magnetic field. The boiler was inadequately wired and wasn't earthed. It was also directly beneath the bath, in the basement. She then told us that her son often got epileptic fits while having a bath, or just afterwards. She couldn't afford to get an electrician in to earth the boiler, but her son's fits went down considerably by having Beacons by the electric meter and around the house."

According to the remote diagnosis Jacqui and David carried out for me, I am very lucky as my house is remarkably free from environmental stress (also lucky their remote tuning doesn't pick up on looming deadline anxieties!). I was told that while an average home can need between three and six products to achieve harmony, I would only need one, to balance a bit of geopathic and geopsychic stress, but it's not essential.

Environmental Harmony provides simple advice for anyone wanting to make their home safer (see below), but one thing Jacqui stresses is to **avoid having digital cordless phones** (analogue ones are better). "They might be convenient, but I would tell anyone with cancer to get rid of them because the waves still come out of the base station, even if you're not using them. The fields can go up through three floors, so anyone living in flats beware. I've been to a house where the noise, registering on our equipment, was so bad that even the pillows were resounding – and the phone wasn't in that room. As soon as it was unplugged, the resounding stopped."

I've heard what these Energy Mixing Beacons do, and seen them (they are handmade blue or green sealed glass bottles containing a natural mineral, crystals and a self-cleansing mechanism) but how do they work? "The cleansing article is made of copper and has an ancient geometric configuration in the middle, which is part of its success when we've processed the mineral. It's a bit like a light bulb," explains David, "you can see the light but not the heat coming from it. This is a frequency that is fed onto the mineral. It creates a field that actually oscillates, quietly brushing your auric field (the electric and magnetic and thermal fields that radiate from the body). The products are the anchors of the energy that they have balanced. Microwave bands and the whole electromagnetic spectrum penetrate the auric field of the body and we have various ways of tackling it. We know that the products correct the magnetic field to magnetic north, this has been measured, but importantly these products are not magnetic at all."

Jacqui and David made their first products in Canada with their partner, nutritional expert Peter Webb. "We made them in jam jars and put them in the basements of Canadian houses," recalls David. "It was an extraordinary thing, but people felt so much better that we realised it wasn't just placebo. "

The most difficult product to develop was the Harmony Token, which is a ceramic disc, containing 2,800 colours to rebuild and repair the body at a cellular level. They are currently testing a cream, containing an organic mineral base used by American Indians for healing.

Some of the techniques Jacqui and David describe sound very unusual but, in the 12 years that Environmental Harmony has been harmonising, their products have been placed in hundreds of homes. There are pages of glowing testimonials covering everything from people's sickness during chemo being relieved, through to aches, children's behavioural problems and even cases of ME and tinnitus disappearing. We at **icon** can't say their methods definitely work, but they can't hurt – and the following tips certainly make a lot of sense.

Reducing manmade electro-magnetic stress in your home

1   Call in an electrician to check your wiring, if your home has not been rewired for more than 20 years.

2   Be aware where you position TVs, hi-fis, computers and battery chargers, as their EMFs can penetrate through walls.

3   Avoid installing a satellite dish on the wall immediately behind the bed area, or make sure the television is earthed.

4   Use battery alarm clocks, instead of electric ones, or keep them at least four feet away from the bed.

5   Do not trail or coil wires under beds and turn off and unplug any equipment immediately behind them (apart from side lights).

6   Avoid placing a bed above fluorescent lights in the kitchen,

as these emit radiation which can cause bed springs to be passive resonators of EMFs.

7 *Do not have the meter and fuse box in the bedroom, or directly above or below the bed areas. This is particularly important in children's rooms.*

8 *If you insist on keeping your microwave, unplug it when not in use and do not put it under the central heating boiler as the microwave radiation may affect the water in your system. Microwaves will also travel into nearby refrigerators and food cupboards, affecting the quality of food. David Broom has Kirlian photography showing how microwaves destroy the energetic aura of even the freshest vegetables; and Eric Kopf in Germany has assembled all German and Russian scientific data on microwaved food showing it is denatured and raises the number of pre-cancerous cells in the human blood stream.*

26 What caused your cancer?
Dowsing for answers
Elizabeth Brown

icon May/June 2004

Our environment is integral to our health and well-being. Our bodies are currently subjected to levels of pollution never before experienced in recorded history. We are exposed to chemical pollution in our water, soil, foodstuffs and manufactured goods, and are surrounded by a complexity of electric, magnetic and electromagnetic fields: computers, domestic appliances, telephones (mobiles and land lines), microwaves, underground and overhead power lines, mobile phone masts, transport systems, hospital equipment, radio and television, radar and satellite. All these factors contribute to a compromised immune system and the subsequent imbalances in our body that result in lethargy, ill health and disease.

It has been established that electromagnetic fields affect our organic tissues – and man-made electromagnetic fields are thousands of times stronger than natural ones. The evidence is rapidly accumulating of the latent harm this unseen environment can cause our mental, emotional and physical health. There is also evidence to suggest that *natural* electromagnetic fields can detrimentally affect our health and well-being.

Elizabeth Brown started as a Geopathic Stress Consultant. She has been in demand for the last few years surveying residential and commercial premises for geopathic stress and electromagnetic pollution, in order to identify the effects they have on the health and well-being of the occupants. She removes or deactivates any detrimental environmental energies and her clients –

according to their testimonials – get better. All this is done by a form of dowsing which is similar to kinesiology, tapping into the information field of the body and its environment.

What is geopathic stress? In simple terms it is the disruption or distortion of the earth's natural electromagnetic field. When this field is in balance it is necessary and restorative to optimal health. When it is corrupted – as it can be by natural geological faults, underground flowing water, mineral deposits, noxious sites and man-made excavations and construction – the changed frequency becomes harmful to our health. This is geopathic stress.

Geopathic stress is not a sickness with its own unique pathology, but it is measurable with Vega and Bio resonance machines. Geopathic stress suppresses the immune function, shutting down the body's natural defence system, thereby facilitating illness. Any natural weaknesses or genetic disorders can be amplified. A study carried out by Dr Eugene Melnikov, Director of the Medical and Ecological Department, St Petersburg, Russia looked specifically at an area covering five square kilometers of interconnecting streets. Every hospital and medical record of those individuals living in the area was checked. Where there was no geopathic stress, little or no occurrence of oncological or other diseases showed. In the geopathically stressed areas, 90 per cent of oncological cases occurred. There was also direct correlation between childhood leukaemia and geopathic stress.

The acceptance of geopathic stress, however, has been marred due to the over-enthusiasm and exaggerated claims of some who attribute all ill-health, disease and accidents to geopathic stress. Brown is convinced through her experience and case studies that *geopathic is only one* of the causative or contributory factors in ill health, and specifically cancer.

Her work has now evolved to embrace all subtle energies. Her dowsing enables her to pinpoint the missing piece of the jigsaw

– whether it be geopathic stress, electromagnetic pollution, toxins in cosmetic or personal care products, environmental pollutants, a nutritional deficiency, subtle energies in the home, or mental and emotional stress – that is the underlying cause of ill health.

Everyone seems to be looking for the mythical one cause of cancer but, during the course of her work, she has come to three very clear conclusions:

- Each case of cancer is as individual as the individuals themselves.

- There is rarely one single cause of cancer, but rather a combination of factors.

- The combination of these factors leads to an imbalance in the body that manifests as cancer.

Each of our bodies is privileged to be unique in its genetic make-up, conditioning and vibrational rate. It is precisely because of this that Brown works to determine the causative, contributory and trigger factors behind each individual's specific cancer. Consider the following:

Sarah requested a residential survey to check for any detrimental environmental energies. She had previously had breast cancer four years before, but was currently in remission. Although 10 years at her current home, her survey request was prompted by the fact that she had never liked going into her bedroom – despite a light and airy room that had undergone complete redecoration. Her unease was justified: Brown identified a geopathic stress line running through the bedroom, with Sarah's bed neatly positioned right in the middle of it. The original cause of the line was geological, but the inherent electromagnetic fields were exacerbated by man-made construction and excavation in the area four to five years before. The timing prompted Sarah to ask whether the geopathic stress was the cause of her cancer. It wasn't, although Brown confirmed that it was certainly a contributory factor through the suppression of the immune system.

Now curious, Sarah wanted to know the key causative factor behind her cancer. After all, how could she — or anyone else who has suffered from cancer — avoid a recurrence without knowing and addressing the root cause? This was really fundamental.

Working through a checklist of possible contributory factors Brown stopped at 'cosmetic products — chemical hair dye carcinogens', but was confused by Sarah's appearance. Her hair, glossy and long, was naturally dark. Brown's question "Have you ever dyed your hair, Sarah?" was greeted by "Oh my God. For four years I dyed my hair blonde, but stopped after the onset of the cancer". The main causative factor in Sarah's cancer was hair dye carcinogens. Further analysis showed that, along with the geopathic stress, deodorant toxins were also a contributory factor. The trigger factor was emotional stress from a difficult relationship with her partner.

The information given to Sarah changed her life. Her understanding of the different factors enabled her to move forward with confidence. She knew what she had to change her life. Rather than battling with an unknown enemy, she felt back in control.

With the fear of the unknown removed she was able to develop positive expectations for the future. This is a vital step because otherwise the fear in itself can become a contributory factor.

Linda also had had breast cancer. For peace of mind she wanted her home checked for anything potentially detrimental to her health and well-being. Also, as a wholistic practitioner, she needed reassurance that her treatment rooms provided the best possible healing environment for her clients. Brown identified and deactivated a geopathic stress line running through her house that was having quite a considerable effect on Linda's health and immune system. This time, however, the geopathic stress was one of *three causative factors* in her cancer. Brown was able to determine that powerful electromagnetic fields at Linda's place of work, coupled with her genetic pre-disposition to cancer were the two other factors. The trigger factor in this instance was confirmed as high levels of emotional stress when Linda was thrust into the role as the main breadwinner of the family, due to her husband's unexpected redundancy.

Again empowered by the information she was given, Linda has reduced her stress levels, underwent a detoxification programme, modified her place of work, and follows a strict health regime to maximise the strength of her immune system. Like Sarah, she now also feels in control of a previously unknown enemy and has the key information to avoid its return.

By knowing the causative, contributory and trigger factors an appropriate course of action, and level of treatment, can be chosen. Brown's contribution is perhaps best summarised by Dr Mark Atkinson of the Harley Street Whole Body Healing Centre "Elizabeth Brown has been gifted an extraordinary ability to get to the heart of an individual's health problem and, more importantly, facilitate the changes required to bring that person back in to harmony again." The changes identified by Brown may be simple, but highly significant, changes in lifestyle.

She currently supports doctors and practitioners to pinpoint the necessary information to help build a totally integrated treatment programme. Whilst the best of orthodox and complementary therapies may ensure that every conceivable step is taken to minimise the possibility of the cancer's return, all the surgery, radiotherapy, chemotherapy, and complementary therapies available will be potentially in vain if the root cause remains unaddressed.

Identification of the cause, therefore, has to be the key to the elimination of cancer.

Geopathic stress in more detail
The earth, like all things living, has an energy field. This energy is partly geomagnetic in composition and partly a force not yet identified by mankind. It radiates from the earth in a system of grid lines relating to the magnetic north and south poles. When in balance the energy is necessary, and restorative, to optimal health. When the natural field is distorted or disrupted – as it can be by natural geological faults, underground flowing water, mineral deposits, noxious sites and man-made excavations and construction – the field becomes harmful to our health. This is geopathic stress.

Geopathic stress suppresses the immune function, shutting down the body's natural defence system, thereby facilitating illness. Any natural weaknesses or genetic disorders can be amplified. The illnesses are often not minor: 70 years of research has shown the correlation between geopathic stress and cancer.

In 1929, German scientist von Pohl proved to the satisfaction of the Central Committee for Cancer Research in Berlin that "one was unlikely to get cancer unless one had spent some time in geopathically stressed places – mainly when sleeping". Then, of course, the human body was not subjected to today's levels of electromagnetic pollution from low level to microwave frequencies, plus the chemical pollution that exists in so many of our foodstuffs, plastics, cosmetics and cleaning products. All these lead to the imbalances in our body that result in cancers. The Committee published von Pohl's findings and today, in some EU countries, planning permission for certain buildings is withheld unless the site has been surveyed for geopathic stress.

Geopathic stress has been found to be the common factor in countless serious, and minor, illnesses, notably those conditions where the immune system is severely compromised: ME or chronic fatigue syndrome; eczema and psoriasis; arthritis; migraine or persistent headaches; glandular fever; insomnia; epilepsy; rheumatism; blood disorders and anaemia; depression; learning and behavioural problems in children. Studies have shown that geopathic stress alters the polarity of the blood, inhibits the blood clotting function, and disrupts electrochemical activity. Geopathic stress also appears to sensitise the body to various electromagnetic fields of other frequencies.

Exposure to geopathic stress might initially manifest as a relentless exhaustion; frequently waking with a feeling of tiredness and a fuzzy head; restless sleep or insomnia; persistent headaches; recurrent colds, viral or fungal infections; depression; heightened allergic responses; and the inability to heal or recover from sickness or respond to treatment. And the common observation shared by countless people prior to the removal of the geopathic stress: 'when spending time away from the home the condition improves or even disappears'. This consistent observation and much published research, has shown that the link between location and sickness is beyond doubt. In all cases of recurring or persistent ill health, geopathic stress should be eliminated early on as a causative factor.

The crucial part that the earth's energy plays in our well-being has been recognised by NASA. During early space missions astronauts suffered from distress symptoms caused by the deprivation of the earth's natural wavelength. In 1952 Professor W O Schumann of Germany identified these waves and, today, Schumann Wave Simulators are installed in manned spacecraft.

27 Disrupting the power stations of brain tumours

Professor Geoffrey Pilkington

icon May 2003

During my career of over 30 years laboratory-based research into the biological nature of brain tumours much knowledge has been gained yet there have been very few, if any, developments which have excited me more than the seemingly bizarre finding that an antidepressant drug may provide an effective way to combat this resistant group of cancers.

The major types of tumours, which begin from the substance of the brain, are known collectively as gliomas. These may arise as high-grade malignancies or may be low grade, benign tumours. Unfortunately the so-called benign tumours frequently develop into malignant tumours with the passage of time. The devastating news that patients with the most malignant form of glioma – known as glioblastoma multiforme - are faced with is that in the absence of treatment they are likely to live for only a few months. Even with surgery, radiotherapy and possibly cytotoxic chemotherapy the five-year survival rate is very poor. The use of cytotoxic drugs in this group of tumours also remains controversial since the modest survival benefit claimed by some workers has to be tempered by the probable reduction in quality of life.

Sadly, despite all the advanced imaging and surgical technology and genetically based approaches to therapy there has been little to encourage either patients or clinicians in the fight against malignant glioma over the past 40 years. Now, following several years' laboratory research, trials have finally begun for anaplastic astrocytoma and glioblastoma multiforme (the two most malignant forms of primary brain tumour in adults) using a drug that has been known to us throughout these past four decades – as an antidepressant!

I was first introduced to the concept of the antidepressant, clomipramine, as a potential anti-cancer agent through a small scrap of University College, London headed paper from Professor David Wilkie. David, who is a well-respected retired Professor, had simply written that he had read my papers on brain tumour cell invasion and thought he had something that might interest me. In short we met and David explained how, through his early studies with yeast cells, he had shown that the tricyclic drug imipramine, and its more active chlorine derivative, clomipramine (or chlorimipramine) influenced energy metabolism and that cancer cells might, at least in theory, be combated by this agent.

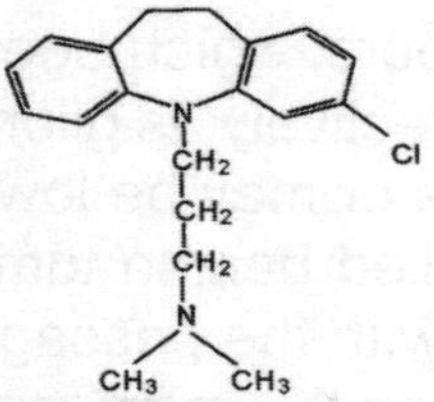

Figure 1 Chemical structure of clomipramine

If clomipramine was able to act selectively on cancer cells due to their compromised respiratory function, as appeared to be the case, then this drug was indeed to be applauded. Clomipramine is one of a group of tricyclic drugs, a name based on their chemical structure (Figure 1). Its major use had been in treatment of obsessive/compulsive and clinically depressed patients. As far as the seemingly strange possibility of treating brain tumours with such an agent was concerned, it did have a number of very attractive features. Notably, after oral administration it is stored in high quantities in both the brain and lung and it has a long half-life of approximately 24 hours, which is increased to 40 hours once metabolised in the body to its by-product, desmethyl clomipramine. The longer the half-life, the longer before the agent will break down. The very fact that the drug crosses the so-called 'blood-brain barrier' (which is formed by specialised blood vessels within the brain) and therefore enters the normal brain is a great advantage in the treatment of brain tumours. Many of the cytotoxic drugs used get into the major mass of the brain tumour by virtue of the fact that the barrier is broken down within the tumour but at the tumour's edge many cancer cells migrate or 'invade' into the normal brain and are protected from these cell-killing drugs by the 'blood-brain barrier'.

We first started to work on the action of clomipramine on brain tumour biopsies in the form of an MSc student project over a 6-month period. Here both the student, Emma Daley, and I were surprised and delighted to note that, while the drug killed cancer cells, in a dose dependant manner, normal brain cells were completely unaffected. We also looked at a number of other agents with a very similar chemical structure notably chlorpromazine (a tranquilizing drug used extensively in the treatment of psychosis) and clofazimine (an anti-leprosy drug) but these either failed to kill tumour cells or caused only reversible damage, killing merely a proportion of component cells of the tumour. On the basis of these early studies I submitted a grant application to the Samantha Dickson Research Trust for funding of a more in-depth analysis of how the drug may work and which tumour types might be sensitive. We were lucky enough to receive three years support from the Trust and recruited the all important help and collaboration of Dr Tim Bates a senior mitochondrial biochemist from the Institute of Neurology in London. After just a few assays where the action of clomipramine was compared with standard inducers of cell death, Tim was just as excited at what he was seeing as we were.

Unlike most cytotoxics, which act by damaging the DNA within the nucleus of the cells, clomipramine acts via cellular respiratory centres, called mitochondria, which are responsible for production of energy for the cell's various activities. The mode of action is therefore, different in that it promotes natural cell death (called apoptosis or programmed cell death) due to compromised respiratory function in cancer cells while leaving normal cells unaffected. In essence, the drug enters the mitochondria, affects complex III of the respiratory chain, reduces oxygen consumption, thereby increasing reactive oxygen species and liberating cytochrome c as a consequence. This, in turn activates a series of enzymes which result in programmed cell death. On the basis of these experimental studies the University of London awarded Emma Daley the degree of Doctor of Philosophy.

Interestingly, Professor John Gordon of the University of Birmingham has recently found clomipramine to have a similar action on lymphoma cells and has also noted that another group of antidepressants, the selective serotonin reuptake inhibitors (SSRIs), appear to elicit similar effects. We have now gone on to assess the effects of other tricyclic drugs including another anti-depressant, which appears to elicit a similar anti-cancer effect to that seen with clomipramine. We have also examined the interaction between clomipramine and anti-convulsants as well as steroids, both of which are commonly prescribed to brain tumour patients. Interestingly the steroid dexamethasone, has an additive effect when used with clomipramine in evoking programmed cell death of brain tumour cells.

Although the clinical trial is still in its infancy, to date, some 300 'anecdotal' cases have been treated. Although the longest standing glioblastoma patients have only been receiving clomipramine for 4.5 years, there have been numerous reports of reduction on tumour mass on MRI scanning, increased survival times, marked clinical improvement and improved quality of life over and above those treated with surgery and radiotherapy alone or with adjuvant cytotoxic chemotherapy. Moreover, benefit to patients who had failed both radiotherapy and cytotoxic chemotherapy, has been apparent.

The side effects are generally mild and include tiredness and dryness of the mouth (which may reduce with time). Since the drug lowers the threshold for seizures in patients whose tumours are likely to give rise to such events, the level of anti-convulsant treatment should be carefully monitored. It is also important for patients to inform their doctors if there are any additional possible side effects such as palpitations or difficulty in passing urine. Patients on drugs known as monoamine oxidase inhibitors will not be allowed to take clomipramine. Since the drug has been widely used over 35–40 years there is more than adequate information on toxicity and therefore a phase I trial was not necessary. Administration is orally as either capsules or tablets but, unfortunately, clomipramine syrup has been recently withdrawn due to low usage. For those patients whose tumours progress despite clomipramine treatment due to a cellular resistance to the drug, we hope that treatment with a second tricyclic anti-depressant or other agents currently under investigation in our laboratories may be possible.

The question arises of when or whether to stop treatment if the tumour shows no clinical or MRI/CT scan based evidence of progression. Unfortunately, at this stage we do not have a real answer but, if patients do come off it, it is recommended that this be done slowly in gradual increments. Our suggestion is, however, to stay on the drug long term and only if neuro-imaging shows sustained and total response in terms of inactivity of tumour should cessation of drug use be considered.

The research work does not end here, however, and I would not claim that clomipramine is in itself a 'gold bullet' glioma cure all. Nor would I claim that it is suitable for the treatment of all brain tumours. Indeed, we are currently exploring ways of enhancing the action of clomipramine and other pro-apoptotic drugs. To these ends we have recently shown that certain enzymes, such as cathepsin L, which are present in high amounts in gliomas and increase with grade of malignancy, protect tumour cells against apoptosis. Therefore, inhibitors of these enzymes may be of clinical use. We are now investigating such inhibitor systems in collaboration with Professor Tamara Lah of the Slovenian National Institute of Biology, Ljubljana. In addition, our studies have gained considerable support from Dr Robert Jones, who has, over the years, made an in-depth study of the role of tricyclic drugs and dietary supplements in the treatment of cancer. Dr Jones reports that the suspicion that certain polyunsaturates participate in the tumour cell killing process indicates that supplementation of clomipramine therapy with omega 3 oils may be of value. In addition, Dr Kathy Aitchison, a consultant psychiatrist and senior lecturer at the Institute of Psychiatry Kings College, London and an expert in tricyclic drug medication, has been of great help in our studies.

Perhaps the most frustrating thing about using a drug such as clomipramine, which is relatively inexpensive and now out of patent, is that the major pharmaceutical companies show little interest in its novel use as an anti-cancer agent. If we could develop a new drug with a similar structure and activity and, more significantly greater marketing potential, we would perhaps be in a better position.

The clinical trial, supported by the Samantha Dickson Research Trust, began in June 2003 at King's College and St Thomas' Hospitals for patients between 16 and 65 years of age with newly diagnosed and histologically verified anaplastic astrocytoma or glioblastoma multiforme. It is hoped that the trial will be extended to other centres in the UK and that if further funding can be provided with support from paediatric oncologists it may be possible to extend the trial to children suffering from brain stem glioma.

28 A new approach to cancer treatment

Dr Robert Jones MA PhD

Robert Jones is a scientist who began cancer research in 1959. He argues that the cancer establishment has not taken new treatments offering hope to many sufferers sufficiently seriously.

Examination of mummified bodies has established that the ancient Egyptians knew forms of cancer. Considering the problem from a philosophical standpoint, it appears odd that no generally effective treatment has been found when temporary regression of malignant disease is a phenomenon, which though rare, is by no means unknown.

Cancer chemotherapy began in the wake of World War II, when American doctors obtained limited success in treating patients with derivatives of highly toxic mustard gas. Since those early days a huge variety of chemical means of inducing the death of cancers in the living body have been devised.

Conventional chemotherapy has for the most part sought to prevent the growth of cancers by using poisons to block the division of cancer cells. Unfortunately maintenance of the mammalian body involves cellular division within all organs, especially the bone marrow and mucosal surfaces of the intestine. The poisons act indiscriminately against normal and cancerous tissues alike, and are responsible for the unpleasant side effects commonly experienced by so many patients. Nature has shown her resentment of the imposition of unnatural forms of cell death by stubbornly refusing to cooperate with clinicians. The underlying strategy is fundamentally flawed, which is why the current impasse prevails.

The basic difficulty has stemmed from ignorance of how tumour cells die. In fact the seeds of understanding were sown centuries ago. Long before the role of bacteria in infection was understood, it had been known that cancers in hosts developing certain kinds of infection, notably erysipelas, underwent regression, usually temporary. In 1891 the American surgeon William Coley recognised the importance of the observations. "Nature often gives us hints to her profoundest secrets," he wrote, "and it is possible she has given us a hint which, if we will but follow, may lead us to the solution of this difficult problem." He treated patients with a mixture of preparations of pathogenic and non-pathogenic bacteria. Unfortunately the responses were highly variable and much too unsuccessful to use clinically. Therapy with mixed toxins remains the province of the truly heroic, determined to hang on to life come what may.

It was not until the 1970s that the destructive changes underlying the few successes Coley reported were at last understood. When tumour-bearing mice were treated with a purified form of a bacterial toxin, it was found that the production of chemical energy within the cancers was rapidly halted. Within a day tumours were quite dead, and sloughed off the bodies of the animals within two weeks. Nature's profound secret was revealed at last; the trick is to disrupt the main source of energy of the malignant cell.

The quest for safe pharmacological alternatives began on a very modest scale. Serendipity ended the search. Anti-cancer activity is present in a number of so-called tricyclic drugs, at least one of which, Largactil, was shown in 1959 to attack energy production in tumours selectively. Most of these drugs act on the brain. In 1990 Dr Riad Mahmud, a diabetologist working in a London teaching hospital passed on experiences gained while working at a hospital in Kuwait in the early 1970s. He had three patients with inoperable cancer of the pancreas, a painful form of cancer with a bad prognosis. Initially he gave promethazine, an anti-histamine and paediatric sedative, by the intravenous route. The drug was followed by calcium, and then given orally every eight hours. One patient died thirteen years later, but not from cancer; in 1990 the other two were still alive. Dr Mahmud was urged to publish, but before the paper could be written he died.

A safe and humane treatment for cancer based on Dr Mahmud's observations and effective in the early stages of disease became available at the end of 1994. Promethazine, the active principle of the therapy, was introduced into clinical practice in 1947 and is long out of patent. In marked contrast with standard cancer drugs, no fatalities appear to have been recorded despite widespread international use.

The first patient to adopt the procedure was a lady in her early forties with breast cancer. Through an administrative failure by the hospital she was made to wait for nine months before receiving specialist attention, by which time her cancer was well advanced. Surgery failed to remove the malignancy completely and chemotherapy produced only a transitory regression. Radiotherapy led to neuritis and caused such intense pain that she sought to have her arm amputated on the affected side. Promethazine brought permanent relief, and two of the four secondaries lodged in the bone disappeared.

Tragically the treatment was stopped prematurely after five months, far too soon. Recommencement produced no advantage, and the patient died eighteen months later. **It cannot be overstressed that, once begun, the treatment has to be continued for at least six months beyond the complete elimination of disease.**

The procedure was published on the Internet in 1996. An updated version together with the scientific rationale is available on www.cancersupportwa.org.au/Spotlight/index.htm A farmer's wife in Western Australia diagnosed with non-Hodgkin lymphoma in 1997 began the new treatment at the age of 55. Eight months later she was declared cancer-free. Unfortunately she too stopped prematurely. Nine months later her condition returned and, as in the previous case, a return to the therapy was ineffective. She underwent a variety of treatments in the hope of regaining sensitivity, including cutting gluten out of the diet. The cancer did become sensitive again but returned once more, and she died five years after the original diagnosis.

Since then a variety of cancers have displayed sensitivity to promethazine, including further cases of non-Hodgkin lymphoma and pancreatic carcinoma, a grade III astrocytoma, a chordoma, stomach cancer, colorectal cancer, Ewing's sarcoma and an instance of breast cancer with secondaries in liver and lung. Although the data are anecdotal and the patients were receiving a wide range of conventional treatments, the common factor has been that improvements began only after the initiation of therapy with promethazine. Even those patients whose cancers failed to regress have enjoyed a better quality of life and prolonged survival.

The health of sufferers has not always improved. Three patients taking high-dose supplements of vitamin E (400, 750 and 1200 units daily) failed to respond, as did others whose disease was seriously advanced. The ability of tumours to accumulate vitamin E has been known since 1940, and the protective effects of the trace nutrient now seem to extend to tumours. More serious is the intractable condition of multi-drug resistance; a single cell clone arising from a mutation caused by orthodox treatment becomes, in effect, immortal.

Simultaneous discovery is rather more common in science than the general public might believe. For a number of years Professor David Wilkie, a geneticist, suspected that the sedative clomipramine might find use against tumours of the brain. The study is still in its early days, but Professor Geoffrey Pilkington together with several clinical consultants has been obtaining encouraging results with these intractable forms of the disease (see Chapter 27).

Unexpected problems have beset introduction of the therapy of cancer with promethazine. Although the cost is less than two pounds a week, patients given the advice may decide not to proceed. Second, the attitude of the medical profession has been consistently indifferent. Letters written to doctors caring for individual patients who are getting better never receive replies; one consultant even went so far as to equate the offered advice with gossip. In sharp contrast, what is remarkable is the willingness of doctors to embark upon clinical trials with newly patented drugs, which more often than not, fail to realise the anticipated success.

Before amalgamating with the Cancer Research Campaign to form Cancer Research UK, the Imperial Cancer Research Fund was sent the rationale for the procedure in 1996. By way of response a senior clinician refrained from comment; the organisation had nobody working in that area, and there were no plans to begin. Approached at the same time, the Cancer Research Campaign preferred to place its faith in molecular biology, and looked to gene therapy to provide the solution to the problem of cancer.

Pharmaceutical companies have shown hardly any interest. Almost all tricyclic drugs are out of patent, so no fat profits can be expected from the introduction of these novel treatments. One manufacturer has argued that it would cost too much to mount a clinical trial for a return expected to be only meagre, though that has not prevented an American company from hiking the price of its generic product up last year from 3 cents to a whopping 31 cents per tablet.

So can a solution to the cancer problem ever emerge? Imagine a cheap and humane self-treatment that works against most cancers, has a good success rate, produces so few side effects that patients can go about their business normally while sustaining the full force of the therapy, causes no deaths and is active against secondary spread. The answer to a prayer, one might think. When used exactly in the manner described, promethazine fulfils these criteria, and is moreover available in most countries without a doctor's prescription. Some, though, conclude that the idea of treating a merciless disease with a paediatric sedative is not to be taken seriously. Proof is urgently needed. Meanwhile no cancer research organisation or commercial enterprise is prepared to undertake a necessary trial. Until cancer patients themselves are prepared to take the initiative, the scourge of cancer will persist unchallenged.

Self-Medication: the Treatment of Cancer with Phenergan?

Introduction: The successful treatment of cancer calls for the total eradication of malignant cells from the body. The therapy aims to destroy both primary and secondary (metastatic) growths by a process of attrition. In marked contrast with conventional treatments the procedure is highly selective; side effects and associated risks are negligible. These are early pioneering days; patients are asked to be realistic and not to allow hopes to rise too high. Although much experience has been incorporated into the following, that there is room for improvement is readily acknowledged. Strict adherence to the advice provided is essential.

No guarantee of a fully successful outcome can be given. Individuals stricken with the disease understandably respond with resentment at the injustice of their dreadful predicaments. As if the initial diagnosis is not bad enough, to be told abruptly that a treatment is not successful is a worse experience that may be lurking in store. Cancer patients deserve respect and dignity; the intention is that the advice provided below should provide a chance of physical healing and spare further anguish. Sincere apologies are made to patients whose malignancies may fail to respond.

Certain drugs acting on the central nervous system possess the additional property of causing injury to tumours by interfering with energy production. Some belong to the large group known a phenothiazines, many of which have been used for half a century. Their diverse uses include the treatment of schizophrenia, nausea and pain. The active drug in this form of cancer treatment is the phenotianzine Phenergan (promethazine), currently used as an anti-histamine, as a paediatric sedative, and to quell travel sickness. An advantage is that its effects on the central nervous system are less marked than those of most other phenothiazines.

This novel and unconventional therapy has several unusual features. First, a new chemotherapeutic target is selected within the cancer cell. Phenothiazines active against cancer trigger a cytotoxic mechanism (necrosis) within the cancer cell itself. The continual state of partial disablement of the power-houses (mitochondria) that supply the malignant cell with much of chemical energy marks the organelles out as its Achilles heel. The intention of the therapy is to intensify this weakness, forcing gradual destruction upon the tumour. In other words, rather than imposing an artificial (and frequently unsuccessful) form of death upon the cell, a natural phenomenon is invoked.

Second, in order to produce its anti-cancer action Phenergan has to be taken according to a specific schedule with the aim of maintaining continuous destructive pressure against malignant growths. Third, provided the primary tumour displays sensitivity to Phenergan, secondary growths will in all probability respond and disappear (see below). Fourth, the treatment is the result of a long investigation standing fully in the tradition of applied medical research.

Logically the next step is to put the therapy to the test in the form of a clinical trial. Despite the impressive weight of supportive scientific evidence (see below), numerous requests and the urgency of the situation, no cancer charity, research council or pharmaceutical company has agreed to do so. Patent cover for Phenergan has long since run out; in consequence the costs are too modest to attract commercial interest. As a point of general advice, although this treatment is no substitute for surgery, Phenergan does seem to be able to reach those parts that the scalpel cannot.

Last but by no means least, the high selectivity of the procedure allows a patient to go about his or her business almost entirely as normal while sustaining the full force of the therapy. There are no hidden snags or sudden ugly costs. If it all sounds too good to be true, that cannot be helped. And if a return to normal life does come about, patients are please requested to give a thought to those enduring the condition which, it is earnestly hoped, has been left behind, and try to interest others who find themselves with cancer in the advice.

Self-Medication – the Schedule:
The treatment is in four parts:
1. First, polyunsaturated fatty acids (the so-called omega-3 fatty acids) or fish origin are needed. Flax oil may also be taken. Patients should aim at a minimum of a gram daily; more is advisable, but the intake can be cut back if bowel looseness is experienced. The purpose of the polyunsaturated fatty acid supplement is to provide cancerous cells with the means to bring about their self-destruction.

2. Second, patients are advised to take 0.5-1.0 grams each of inositol and choline daily. These are naturally-occurring substances normally available from health stores. Some authorities recommend inositol hexaphosphate (IP_6), which contains only 23% inositol and has the disadvantage of forming insoluble precipitates with calcium within the bowel. It may also be more expensive than inositol itself.

   If possible patients should begin to take nutritional supplements, especially polyunsaturated fatty acids, several days before starting with Phenergan.

3. Third, certain micro-nutrients are recommended with the intention of protecting the white cells of the blood against rare side-effects (blood dyscrasias). A multi-vitamin/ mineral preparation containing the recommended dietary allowance (RDA) of copper (2.5mg), manganese (4mg), zinc (15mg) and selenium (50mcg, or 0.05mg) is necessary. Minor devi-

ations from these amounts, which should be taken daily, are unimportant. Vitamin supplements in excess of RDA values, especially vitamin C (RDA 60mg) and vitamin E (RDA 10-15 international units [iu]; see later), must be avoided as far as possible.

All supplements should be continued for the entire duration of the therapy.

4. Fourth, treatment is initiated by taking Phenergan as a 50mg dose one evening at retiring. It is necessary to continue eight hours later on the following day with 25mg, with 25mg every eight hours thereafter until an adequate period of time has elapsed *after* the last traces of disease have disappeared. At present that period is arbitrarily put at six months, but should be extended if any doubt exists over the elimination of disease.

In most countries Phenergan can be freely purchased in the form of 10mg and 25mg tablets; other phenothiazines are available only on prescription. Formulations in which the drug is provided in conjunction with other drugs are not recommended.

Success depends on maintaining continuous pharmacological pressure against the cancer throughout the entire period of treatment. Even if the treatment fails to half the progress of disease, Phenergan can enhance quality of life and extend survival. In other words, the therapy places the patient in a no-lose situation.

Contra-Indications: Cancer patients are unlikely to benefit from this treatment if:

1. Steroids are being administered in high doses. Interference with anti-cancer activity is, however, unstable, and therapy with Phenergan can be commenced three days after cessation of steroids.

2. There has been brief or intermittent exposure to phenothiazines or to certain chemically-related drugs after the onset of disease; this, it might be added, would be unusual.

3. Certain analgesics classified as non-steroid anti-inflammatory drugs (aspirin, ibuprofen, diclofenac, etc) are being taken. Here the advice is to wait for a week before commencing.

   Serious pain calls for professional attention. Paracetamol in moderation is suitable; so are opiates (for example, morphine) given on prescription. Provided the pain is not too severe, electrical stimulation with a TENS device (transcutaneous electrical nerve stimulation) can provide a limited measure of relief.

4. The patient is deficient in essential fatty acids. This an uncommon condition of which scaly skin, especially on the backs of the hands, can be an indicator.

   Polyunsaturated fatty acids are micro-nutrients and are required for normal health. Those which participate in the process of tumour destruction are thought to belong to the so-called omega-3 series, and have yet to be identified.

5. There is dietary supplementation with vitamin E.

   The question of vitamin E calls for special mention. Most diets already contain amounts adequate for a healthy life style. For individuals free from cancer dietary supplementation is highly beneficial, offering protection not only against the development of malignancy but also against coronary heart disease. Unfortunately it might be that the same beneficial properties are exploited by cancerous growths, which accumulate vitamin E as protection against successful therapy. Many dietary schedules drawn up expressly for cancer patients include substantial amounts of vitamin E. I personally question the wisdom of these recommendations.

Several patients on vitamin E supplements (400-1200iu daily) failed to respond to Phenergan. Current advice is therefore to stop supplementation immediately and to wait 7-10 days. Likewise, selenium supplementation above the RDA is not recommended.

6. Multi-drug resistance (*mdr*) can arise during radiotherapy or treatment with certain cytotoxic drugs. It is not generally recognised that a mutation in a cancerous cell may result in a partial or complete disablement of the cytotoxic mechanism. Clones of these mutant cells grow rapidly and are generally insensitive to therapy.

7. The disease is prostatic or mesothelioma. Several cases of the former and a single instance of the latter failed to respond to Phenergan. With mesothelioma there is a chance that *mdr* was present, but perhaps not with the cancers of the prostate. Anyone with either condition is welcome to try the therapy, but should be warned that the chances of response do not seem to be good.

The success of this treatment depends on various factors, of which one is the state of advancement of the disease. No matter how hopeless the situation may appear, a positive response to Phenergan is not out of the question. **Under no circumstances should Phenergan treatment be discontinued prematurely; if treatment is interrupted before the growth is wholly eradicated the treatment will have no anti-tumour effect the second time round.** No reason is known for this peculiar behaviour, and no means of resensitisation is known at the present time. The maxim is: if in doubt, don't quit out.

In view of the serious consequences of premature discontinuation, if a marked improvement is maintained after a few weeks patients would be well advised to purchase sufficient Phenergan to last for two or three months in case procurement becomes difficult.

Response to Therapy: A general improvement in terms of weight gain, improved sleep, restored appetite and general well being should be perceptible at least by the end of the first week. Lessening of pain is an encouraging sign, but where there is involvement of bone several weeks may pass before relief is noticed. A record of body weight should be kept. The advice on offer is gentle and humane; for those with experience of the fiercer forms of chemotherapy and radiotherapy the difference will come as a welcome surprise.

Side Effects: The commonest of these is sedation; on the whole patients do not find the experience unpleasant, but driving a car and using machinery or sharp tools are not recommended, at least for the first fortnight. Some patients are quite unaffected. Drowsiness in the first few days after commencing Phenergan normally lasts not more than a week. In a few cases sedation persists; more rarely patients may become excited or 'twitchy', as the experience has been described. In these instances the dosage can be halved, with a 10mg tablet every 8 hours and an extra 10mg at night, making a total of 40mg.

Few patients experience difficulty with Phenergan therapy. Two patients have maintained themselves on the full schedule for over three years; one experienced a modest gain in weight. Only one patient found the therapy insupportable, but he responded to every medication in the same manner. There are very small chances that jaundice may develop within a few days, or that the white cell count may fall (leucopenia or agranulocytosis) after 4-6 weeks. The former can be recognised by a yellowing of the features, the latter by sore throat. Thrombocytopenia (fall in platelet count) is again highly unlikely, and may be indicated by unexplained bruising or cuts bleeding for longer than usual. In these instances medical attention should be sought immediately. To date none of these symptoms has arisen among cancer patients taking Phenergan.

Patients with breast cancer who find themselves suffering from radiation-induced peripheral neuritis may find that Phenergan will clear the condition up permanently.

Duration of Treatment and Outcome: Very reasonably, patients may ask whether their particular form of disease is likely to respond to the self-medication procedure described here. The therapy takes advantage of a metabolic weakness common to all malignant tissues so far examined; in theory, then, all cancers should be amenable to treatment. Forms of the disease which have displayed sensitivity include non-Hodgkins lymphoma, breast cancer with secondaries, glioblastoma, a chordoma, colorectal cancer and cancer of the oesophagus, both with secondaries. Whether a favourable outcome ensues depends basically on the circumstances of the patient. Early presentation is helpful. On the basis of previous experience the chances seem to be about fifty-fifty. Other factors which might affect the outcome have been discussed above. What is certain is that unless the therapy is started, it has absolutely no chance of succeeding.

It might be added that it is not considered likely that there will ever be a "cure" for cancer in the fond sense of journalists. Whether all the problems recognised here can be overcome is impossible to say. What is sure is that until the principle of destroying cancer by selectively disrupting energy metabolism within malignant cells is accepted by the scientific establishment, which at present appears unlikely, the merciless toll will continue.

The effects of the therapy should be monitored by any means available. Even a dressmaker's tape measure and a little native wit can provide useful information. The results of scans should be interpreted with care. If therapy is commenced between scans, it should be borne in mind that shrinkage may be offset by tumour growth prior to commencement of therapy. The temptation is to delay in order to make comparisons between the effects of different treatments is to be avoided.

The therapy works slow; just how long it will be necessary to keep taking Phenergan will depend, among other factors, on the extent of the disease when treatment is started and on the state of nutrition. It may be necessary to stay with Phenergan for two years or more, especially where there are secondary deposits in the bone.

Precautions: A leaflet is provided with the Phenergan packet; the advice given should be read and, apart from discontinuation, adhered to. Alcohol does not interfere with the anti-cancer action, but abstinence is advised. Exposure to ultraviolet light and sunlight, especially sunbathing, are to be avoided as far as possible. The group of drugs known as monoamine oxidase inhibitors must not be taken in conjunction with Phenergan.

Relationship of the Patient with the Doctor and Cancer Specialist: Cancer is a serious disease and should at all times be regarded accordingly. *The help and support of medial advisers is valuable and must at all costs be enlisted and retained.* Being secretive is discourteous; keeping your oncologist fully informed is essential, and may stimulate genuine interest and additional sympathy. The patient who manages best is sufficiently brave to face the future with equanimity. Accurate reports of progress need to be requested. Tumour regression is always welcome, but even if the news is not good the therapy should not be abandoned.

If attempts are made to dissuade, it may be asked what the dangers of the treatment with Phenergan are perceived to be: reassurance that the risks are very small is likely to be given. This is a procedure with a firm scientific base. Reference can be made to "Successful Cancer Therapy with Promethazine: the Rational," published in *Medical Hypotheses 46, 25029 (1996).* Further evidence can be found in *Notes on the Treatment of Cancer with Low-Dose Phenotiazines with Special Reference to Promethazine,* currently available on the Spotlight section of the Cancer Support Association of Western Australia. (There are plans to move it to Research). The site address is www.cancersupportwa.org.au. It is necessary to click on the Figure in the text to ensure that the document prints out completely.

Orthodox Treatment and Self-Medication: In England doctors make great efforts to sustain hopes of remission, and are the beneficiaries of measures of deep faith from their patients. Optimism is seen as a valuable asset. An understandable reluctance exists to tell a patient that a condition is incurable, a shattering experience for which few are prepared. Self-delusion, though, is dangerous. Patients have turned self-medication down because they are unaware of the gravity of their situations. In Australia patients are often told there is no chance of recovery. Faced with the inevitable, a common response has been to accept the advice on offer on the understanding there can be no guarantee of permanent benefit.

In some countries there may be less time for deceptive sympathy, and the message can be blunt and uncompromising. Too often patients may be lulled into a dangerous sense of false security by a favourable report of tumour shrinkage and cannot accept the significance of a subsequent relapse. Remissions from conventional treatment are not always permanent. In addition it is not generally understood that once secondary growths become established, chances of recovery with orthodox treatment are remote. On the other hand, when a cancerous cell migrates and establishes itself elsewhere in the body there is no reason why its genetically-determined properties should undergo change. Secondaries originating from Phenergan-sensitive primary growths generally regress and disappear. Experience to date indicates that when the therapy is sufficiently prolonged, relapses do not occur.

Alternative Approaches: Modern medicine is often miraculous. Antibiotics, transplants, open-heart surgery, joint replacements come to mind. Unhappily the conventional treatment of cancer has not kept pace with other advances in healthcare. The failure of medicine opens the door to the glib operator anxious to line his pockets at the expense of the desperate.

Critics of alternative treatments are right to point out that claims of success are never substantiated and that the methodology is never divulged. In stark contrast the scientific evidence in support of Phenergan is in the public domain (see above).

There is a belief that the treatment of cancer with phenothiazines amounts to alternative medicine, fringe medicine. Nothing could be further from the truth. Sometimes one can sympathise with the opposition of doctors to complementary practices, especially when patients and their families are sometimes charged formidable sums for worthless advice and/or nostrums. The more expensive a treatment or preparation is, the greater the need for sceptiscm. Some complementarists are honest enough to admit they offer only palliation, but understandably patients and their families expect more and are often unwilling, unable even, to accept reality.

Here the situation is totally different. Your doctor is unlikely to have heard of the therapy, and may be sceptical. In these circumstances the only question one can reasonably expect to have answered if whether or not harm is likely to ensue. Phenergan was introduced into medical practice as long ago as 1947; most unusually, not a single fatality therefrom has been reported.

In this materialistic age there is a general feeling that everything must have its price. In stark contrasts with private clinics and a majority of alternative approaches, no fee has ever been charged. Patients are expected to meet the modest costs (currently under £2 a week in the UK) of their treatment on their own. Some have mistakenly concluded that advice which costs nothing must by definition be worthless. They have later found themselves to have taken an expensive stance.

Action: If, after reading the above, uncertainty persists, the question remains: what is there to lose? **Now** is the time to decide whether or not to go ahead, and if so, to make plans this very moment. Experience has shown that when the outcome is unfavourable, a point of no return is reached when nothing more can be done. What is certain is that the sooner the treatment begins, or, put another way, the smaller the tumour burden is, the quicker the patient may become cancer-free. Delay confers no advantage whatsoever. The big errors that cancer patients commonly make are to believe that time is on their side and to adopt a wait-and-see attitude. **Nothing could be more mistaken**. Time is never on the side of the cancer patient. The overriding aim must, as a matter of pressing urgency, be to begin as soon as possible to get well gain.

Once more, then: What is there to lose?

29 Photodynamic therapy

Chris Woollams

Will natural, non-toxic agents see the light of day?

Smart bombs
Historically, chemotherapy has had its critics because the chemotherapy agents were too general. They caused disruption in the copying process of cells and so would most disrupt rapidly dividing cells, which of course include cancer cells. Unfortunately, a lot of other cells divide during the chemotherapy period. Result, many of the bad guys were killed off, along with too many good cells as well. Worse, there was no guarantee the chemical agent had destroyed all the cancer cells rather than most. Leave just one healthy cancer cell behind and the potential is there for multiple division and reoccurrence of cancer.

Nowadays scientists are developing 'smart' chemical agents, the sorts that target some physical property unique to a cancer cell – for example its unique enzymes or DNA makeup. After all, if the American military can target a single building in a whole city with a cruise missile, why can't cancer scientists target unique cancer cells amidst a body of otherwise healthy cells?

Interestingly, the era of chemotherapy may be passing already. Only recently the prestigious MD Anderson Cancer Center in Houston stated that all the exciting developments in cancer treatment were in areas other than chemotherapy.

Light relief – Photodynamic Therapy (PDT)
Photodynamic Therapy historically used a chemical agent that

selectively attached to cancer cells. When light of a certain wavelength or frequency was shone on the agent, it excited the agent's atoms encouraging them to offload electrons to any oxygen molecules in the localised vicinity. These then became 'singlet oxygen', highly unstable free radicals.

In turn these oxidised any molecule they came into contact with. And since the original agent was, by now, either attached to, or inside, the cancer cell, the host was destroyed.

The Lancet (December 2000 – Professor Hopper; University College, London Hospital, NHS Trust) stated: "PDT is a minimally invasive treatment with great promise in malignant disease. It can be applied before, or after, chemotherapy, ionising radiation, or surgery, without compromising these treatments or being compromised itself. Unlike radiotherapy and surgery, it can be repeated many times at the same site. Response rates and the durability of response with PDT are as good as, or better than, those with standard locoregional treatments. Furthermore there is less morbidity and better functional and cosmetic outcome".

Lest you have never heard of PDT and/or think it is some sort of new and probably flaky cancer treatment, please be clear.

The technology is supported by over 100 years of research and development; there have been approximately 3500 scientific reviews and articles and there are currently several hundreds of universities and top cancer clinics from New York to Russia seeking to develop and improve this treatment. (Try the Internet site www.medline.com and type in PDT, for example.)

PDT can be applied before or after chemotherapy, radiotherapy or surgery, without compromising these treatments or being compromised itself.

Unlike radiotherapy or surgery, it can be repeated many times at the same site.

Response rates and the durability of response with PDT are as good as, or better than, those with standard loco-regional treatments.

Furthermore, there is less morbidity and a better functional and cosmetic outcome.

PDT – origins
PDT has been around for a century; indeed Neils Finsen won a Nobel Prize in 1903 for using light treatment to cure lupus.

In 1904 the first recorded cure of a cancer took place in Germany, a basal cell carcinoma of the lip.

However the over-excitement of the pharmaceutical and medical establishments for dry based chemotherapy saw PDT put on the 'back burner' until the mid-1970s when a doctor in Buffalo, NY developed a chemical agent and used it to treat cancer. The original agent was developed by Dr Thomas Doherty and received FDA approval as 'Photofrin'. This particular agent was derived from blood, usually pigs' blood.

PDT – classic limitations
As with chemotherapy, the treatment is only as good as the chemical agent. Photofrin is a porphrin and porphrins do selectively attach to cancer cells. Sometimes, in some cases up to the 25 per cent level, the agent attaches to healthy cells and all (bad and good) are killed when the localised area is sensitised by light. The quest over the last thirty years has been to find better, more selective agents.

Another limitation historically, has been the need to have the cancer in a position where light could activate the agent accumulated in the cancer cells. So, for example, work with brain tumours was confined to moments when the skull had been opened up.

The other implication of this 'direct action' was that cancer cells not in the direct line of fire escaped. Thus early procedures where the norm was to treat tumours that were 'seen', often omitted dealing with any secondaries or colonies of cancer cells that had not been spotted in other areas of the body.

Early agents were also slow, both to reach cancer cells and then to clear out of the body afterwards. Photofrin could take two to four days to successfully attach to the cancer cells, and up to 30 days to clear the body. Another agent currently used in the UK, Phoscan, has similar problems. If the agents stay in the body then the patient has to avoid light, for example bright sunlight that could photosensitise them, even 25 days later.

Developments at the speed of light
PDT is improving all the time and the work is gathering pace because the agents and the technology are both improving. You can easily trawl the Internet and find clinics in the USA that use it. The crucial issue in the USA for example, is FDA approval of the photodynamic agent. The FDA tend to prefer single agents rather than complex mixes.

Only recently the team at the Johann Wolfgang Goethe University in Frankfurt treated five liver cancer patients with an agent called SQN400. All had colorectal cancers that had spread to the liver; three of the five were clear of cancer three months later.

In April 2003, **icon** reported on a trial at the Gray Cancer Institute in Middlesex and sponsored by Cancer Research UK. The trial, reported in the journal *Cancer Research*, used a dye combined with plant hormones. When they shone red light on the cells with the dye, the dye 'shattered' and provided chemicals toxic to the cell.

Professor Peter Wardman, who led the study for Cancer Research UK, drew attention to the problem of low oxygen in the cancer cells. The problem with PDT historically was that it worked by activating localised oxygen to produce singlet oxygen, which destroyed the cells. But in most tumours there are low oxygen conditions. Wardman's method uses molecules of plant hormones to attack cancer cells instead. *" Overcoming this oxygen problem is a major challenge in cancer therapy. So far we have shown this works in dishes, but because both the dye and the plant hormone are known to be non-toxic in man, we are hopeful that we can quickly translate this treatment into clinical reality."*

In Russia there is much work on PDT currently. In one company, Rada Pharma, scientists and pharmacists have developed a triple ingredient agent based on algae and chlorophyll, called radachlorin. They are currently investigating it in trials as the nature of the agent allows light of the infrared range to be used to sensitise the agent. This would enable the body to be harmlessly penetrated by the light and so deep-seated tumours could be attacked. In the UK, The Dove Clinic has been working with PDT for some time.

Algae and chlorophyll
It has long been known that the chlorophyll molecule in plants resembles that of haemoglobin in animals. They are structurally similar, the main difference being an iron atom at the centre of haemoglobin, but a magnesium atom in chlorophyll.

Both are crucial in the oxygenation process in an organism.

In plants, sunlight energises the chlorophyll causing oxygen production, a totally natural process.

Populations that consume large amounts of green plants and have lots of sunlight (for example, Mediterranean cultures, or the sun belt in the USA) get less cancers, and it is known that longer wavelength UV plays some part in this.

Some 'diet' therapies involving barley grass, spirulina or wheat grass in part attribute their success to the oxygenating benefits of chlorophyll.

Russian research has looked into chlorophyll, algae and bacteriochlorophyll, the latter being a red type of chlorophyll sensitive to light in the infrared range. This is important because such infrared light can penetrate deeper into the body and sensitise the agent in 'deep seated' tumours.

With the Russian agent, the wait time is claimed to be only hours after infusion intravenously before light treatment can be used. And within 36 hours there is no sensitivity to light as the agent has been eliminated from the skin.

Light Fantastic or Optical Illusion?
Bill Porter is a trained doctor and ophthalmologist. In 1998 he was retired and living in Ireland when his wife was diagnosed with breast cancer. The orthodox treatment suggested typically included surgery, radiotherapy and chemotherapy. When I visited them in spring 2004 she had still had none of these. Instead she wanted to be treated in a non-toxic way and Porter used his knowledge and experiences to look into possible treatments. Because of his own work with light and lasers he became particularly interested in photodynamic therapy.

Porter is a quietly charming man, determined to help his wife but now also to pass on what he has discovered. Unfortunately he has a 'bit of history'. He prefers not to go back to the USA because of an alimony battle with an ex-wife. Worse, he was 'struck off' as an ophthalmologist for leaving a US patient, although he claims his divorce and other factors meant he decided to go and work in The Middle East leaving all his former patients in the hands of his previous colleagues, and the first he heard of any problems was a few years after being struck off!

Who knows?
When his wife was first ill he needed someone to officially treat her and tied up with a local Irish doctor, someone he has since not worked with for several years. However, in the Summer of 2004 they have both been the subject of vicious press attacks, although the detail of the actual accusations related more to his

previous doctor partner. Press reports described them jointly as 'Sickos' *(sic)* for treating vulnerable patients with alternative and expensive cancer treatments. The Garda came to Porter's clinic and took all his files, computers and even the Internationally certified and approved infra-red bed he used.

So what prompted these attacks??
In the last couple of years Porter had managed to lay his hands on some of the Rada Pharma agent. He felt it was good, but still had problems. So he turned to yet another Irish doctor, this time also a pharmacologist, Dr Tom Clearey, and together they specified, had made, registered and patented in the UK, their own agent – Photo Flora. This of course in turn prompted the competitive wrath of, and falling out with, the Russians!! There is big money at stake here.

And Porter opened a new clinic himself, but this time with Dr Clearey admitting and monitoring the patients. And he was getting results. He happily put me in touch with an Australian gentleman who had previously had standard PDT with no improvement, but almost a year ago, a course of this new agent had seen vast improvement in his health – despite a grade 4 diagnosed brain tumour, similar to that of my daughter. In fact the patient is now back on the golf course for the first time in five years.

Interestingly, Porter is very balanced about the commotion going on around him. He feels he has made errors of judgement but that this should not detract from the power of the agent he developed for his wife.

Porter believes we are only at the beginning of this type of therapy, and we are on our way to developing natural, non-toxic plant agents that are far more selective in targeting cancer cells, whilst also being eliminated from the body quickly after treatment. Hence he is not surprised he has been so viciously attacked in Eire, home to so many Pharmaceutical companies. His natural agent would be a cheap, non-toxic replacement for many of their drugs.

Porter sees it as absolutely no coincidence that the haemoglobin and chlorophyll molecules are so structurally similar, nor that agricultural communities who eat more 'green' foods and live out of doors more, develop less cancers.

Dr Clearey's and Bill Porter's Photo Flora is based on spirulina. This natural agent circulates easily in the blood system, without toxic effect, because of its similarity to haemoglobin.

The cancer cell, which produces its energy without oxygen in a fermentation process, is acidic and negatively charged. Because the energy process is less efficient than that of a normal cell, and because cancer cells divide so rapidly, a large amount of 'fuel' is required. In a cancer cell, this 'fuel' is glucose.

The success of this agent is, they claim, that it 'acts' like glucose and so gains easy entry into the cancer cells.

Glucose is normally carried across cell membranes by lipoproteins found in the blood. The agent is also carried this way.

But two other factors make it stick uniquely inside a cancer cell. First, normal cells are slightly alkaline, but by contrast the acidity in a cancer cell disengages the agent from the lipoprotein. Second, the agent has two positive charged areas and thus energetically binds to the negatively charged elements in the unique power stations of the cancer cell.

Meanwhile, the risk of binding to healthy cells falls from about 25 per cent (Photofrin) to less than 3 per cent, so Porter claims, because this new agent specifically 'avoids' healthy cells that are alkaline and not negatively charged. So the very structure and properties of the cancer cell cause the agent to be absorbed uniquely by them. No resistance builds up to it over time either, so repeated sessions can be used.

More remarkably, Porter is now finding that a version of Photo Flora can be taken orally, using drops under the tongue.

Porter calls his therapy **Cytoluminescent Therapy** rather than PDT. Now what did Shakespeare say about a rose? Patients may take the 'green liquid' for a month or just three days depending upon the level of activity required. Then comes the photosensitising treatment, which looks like a giant sunbed! Not only is this slightly less stressful, but it allows build up of the agent throughout the body and he is actually finding that luminescence occurs — releasing oxygen and killing cancer cells — even before the treatment starts!

Light of the correct wavelength is then shone on the body to sensitise the agent. But unlike traditional PDT, the effect is not localised but totally systemic, throughout the body. A major difference and a huge breakthrough since, through other laser techniques, Porter has shown that cancer tumours are rarely confined to one place. More often than not 'hot spots' occur throughout the body.

An added bonus he claims is that the cytoxic effects of the agent and the CLT tend to cause coagulation in the blood vessels that feed the tumour, cutting off its supply of nourishment.

And finally, it would seem that although the death of the cancer cell occurs from 'within', the initial breakdown of the tumour releases inactive cancer cells into the bloodstream that are mopped up by the immune system. This stimulates the immune system to recognise a better level of rogue cells everywhere.

Red light
All this seems too good to be true, and Porter is now looking at other worldwide locations to fulfil his dream. But the truth of CLT and this UK patented agent runs in parallel with B-17, Metabolic Therapy, Gerson etc etc. We cancer researchers, you patients, anybody genuinely responsible and interested in developing life saving cancer treatments: We all need accurate, unbiased results, not hearsay and anecdote.

Porter claims Harvard University Medical School has monitored his treatment and Dr Donald J Burke has described it as 'a quantum leap', with recommendations to Harvard, MIT and Tufts to also conduct trials. However Porter wants to conduct his own clinical trials, and is talking to clinics all over the world about CLT usage and such trials. We wait with interest.

The Dove Clinic in UK is planning to use PDT (CLT) using this new agent, Photo Flora.

Green light
Whatever the outcome with Russian agents, Porter, James Bond, whoever, one thing is for certain: All over the world laboratories are looking for a similar agent – natural, non-toxic, quick to act and to leave the body, working systemically on surface and deep-seated tumours etc etc; and if it can be developed we just could be on our way to a cheap cure.

One thing is for sure, whatever the outcome for Porter and Dr Clearey, the Garda have certainly not stopped this agent from seeing the light of day.

30 Dendritic cell therapy vaccines
A promising new approach to the treatment of cancer

Dr Julian Kenyon

icon May/June 2004

During the last 10 years there has been a rapidly increasing understanding of immune surveillance and appreciation of the mechanisms by which tumours escape its notice. This has led to the development of promising new strategies against cancer, of which the most exciting and consistently successful are dendritic cell therapy vaccines.

The importance of the inter-action between the immune system and cancer cells was recognised in the 1890s by a doctor in New York called William Coley, who used streptococcal cultures (bacterial cultures) to treat patients with advanced carcinomas and sarcomas. These attempts to activate general immunity led to clinical responses and in some cases of Coley's patients, complete remissions, which were long lasting. More recently, antibodies and T-cells (a particular sub-set of white cells that identify tumour antigens these are the proteins on the surface of tumours) have been isolated from patients with cancer. It is clear that the immune system is capable of recognising tumour cells. Cellular immunotherapy or dendritic cell therapy vaccines consists of giving the patient cells that stimulate anti-tumour activity in the patient. The aim is to harness potent immunological weapons to destroy cancer cells.

My interest in this area started over 15 years ago when I was in California, registering our research Charity as a 'for non-profit organisation' in the USA. I was working with the Institute of Noetic Sciences and at that time they were compiling a book entitled 'Spontaneous Remission in Cancer'. I read the proofs of this book, which extended to well over 1,000 pages and is sadly now out of print. I was amazed to find that spontaneous remission has been reported in the medical literature for practically every kind of known cancer and indeed sarcomas in some cases. The most common cancers to spontaneously remit are leukaemias. The remission is nearly always associated with a major infection of some sort. What is clear is that the immune response to an infection, be it bacterial or viral, is similar to an effective immune response against a tumour, and this type of immune response is called a cell-mediated immune response and is predominantly executed by sub-sets of so-called T-(Thymic) white cells. The essential feature of this process is that the T-cells specifically recognise a protein on the surface of a bacteria or a virus in the case of infections, and in the case of tumours specific proteins on the surface of tumours. The T-cells then home-in on the cancer cells or the infecting organism and destroy these cells specifically, without attacking normal cells. This kind of immune surveillance happens in us all the time. One would therefore expect evidence that in people whose immune surveillance was poor, who therefore had low cell mediated immune function, then they should have an increased incidence of cancer. There have been a number of prospective studies following populations over 10 years that show just this and that people with poor cell mediated immunity have, in round figures, a 50 per cent more chance of developing cancer over a 10 year period, in comparison to those people who have good cell mediated immunity. As a civilisation this is a hugely important finding, because our cell mediated immune function, as a civilisation, is generally getting poorer, largely due to the effects of industrial and atmospheric pollution, which tends to push the immune function away from an adequate cell mediated immune response towards an overly active antibody response, and therefore increased incidence of allergies, which is what one finds in the developed world.

Soon after my work in California I came across a patient who consulted me whose story was so remarkable that I've never forgotten it. He was an Italian waiter who had smoked all his life. He had advanced lung cancer. He came to ask me whether I could help him. In the event I could only offer palliative approaches and I was unable to help, but in the course of the history taking, he said that his elder brother had also had lung cancer and had been a smoker all his life. What's more, his brother went for surgery to attempt to remove his lung cancer, but it was found that it was inoperable. Following the operation his brother was sewn up with non-absorbable stitches, extending right from the back of one side of his chest round through to the front. Post-operatively, every site where the stitches went through the skin, became infected and developed into a whole line of large abscess. His brother became extremely ill and it was feared that he would die. What in fact happened was that he recovered, his lung cancer went into complete remission and his brother is now still alive and still smoking. I decided to look into this area further and managed to obtain supplies of a modern version of William Coley's bacterial vaccines. I tried a course of such vaccines injected under the skin in a patient 7 years ago who had mesothelioma of the pleura, a malignant disease of the lining of the lungs caused by asbestos, which is uniformly fatal. This man was in his mid-60s and had a prognosis of less than 6 months. This patient of mine is still alive and well today. He is playing golf and he remains in complete remission. Therefore my interest in this field increased and we now use dendritic vaccines in a wide range of cancers, with encouraging results.

The immune response to cancer
So-called cytotoxic T-lymphocytes are one of the critical effector cells that are able to destroy tumour cells. Receptors on the surface of T-cells recognises proteins called tumour associated antigens on the surface of tumours. However, the process is complex and in order for the T-cell to become activated, it must recognise the tumour associated antigen and it must have a co-stimulatory signal in order to kill off a cancer cell, as in the

absence of this the T-cells become tolerant to the antigen and the tumour continues to grow. The cellular orchestraters of this T-cell activation are antigen presenting cells which are called dendritic cells that possess a remarkable ability to stimulate the immune response. Under the microscope, these cells are about the same size as the average white cell and have long finger-like processes which often divide and it is on these processes that tumour associated antigen is carried and then presented to T-lymphocytes and in that process the co-stimulatory signal is provided and the T-cells recognise the particular antigen presented to them and then go the tumour bearing that antigen and if all goes well, will kill the tumour cells. Dendritic cells are present throughout the body but are particularly prevalent in the skin. This is therefore why in dendritic cell therapy vaccinations some of the injections need to be given into the skin, that means intra-dermal as opposed to under the skin (subcutaneous). This is absolutely critical and is an important reason why some dendritic cell therapy vaccines fail, simply because the injections are given subcutaneously and not into the skin.

In order to make a dendritic cell therapy vaccine, tumour associated antigen needs to be obtained. This can be either from a biopsy of the tumour or part of a specimen removed at operation. Or, it can be obtained from the urine during any treatment programme which destroys tumour cells, such as chemotherapy, or in our case at our clinic, we use high dose intravenous vitamin C and Ukraine (Majus and Thiotepa). In conventional chemotherapy maximal tumour cell death occurs from one day to six days after a chemotherapeutic dose. It is during the first two days of this that the patient is instructed to save their urine and by a special filtration process saving molecules of a particular molecular weight, we are able to isolate tumour antigen specific to that particular patient and use this in order to make a dendritic cell therapy vaccine. Oddly enough, our dendritic cell therapy vaccines made from tumour associated antigen derived from the urine in this way, seem to be more effective than vaccines made from biopsies or part of a tumour removed at operation. It's unclear why this is the case, perhaps when tumour antigen is obtained from the urine it is processed in some way in the body, which makes the tumour antigen more immunologically available. This is called immunogenicity, and increasing the immunogenicity of tumour associated antigen is fundamental to this process, as it makes it more likely that T-lymphocytes will recognise this tumour associated antigen as being foreign and will attack it.

Our dendritic cell therapy vaccine programmes take 3 months and involves nearly 50 intradermal and some subcutaneous injections, which the patient can self-administer. We also, in the first part of the programme, use heat shock proteins, our favourite is heat shot protein 70. Heat shock proteins are released during infections and give a switch-on signal to the immune system. We do this in order to have immune surveillance operating maximally. We look for re-actions after the heat shock proteins have been injected and patients should feel ill for a day, have a red swollen area around the site of the injection and our findings are that the bigger these reactions are, then the more effective the vaccine. The worst kind of situation is where the patient has no reaction whatsoever to the vaccine and therefore in these situations the immune system is unresponsive. There are a range of other complicated factors, many of which we don't yet understand, that attenuate the effect of dendritic vaccines.

Clinical studies
There are many hundreds of papers on dendritic cell therapy vaccines in the medical literature. The numbers are increasing all the time. Also the cancers involved are extending. The first dendritic cell therapy vaccines were used in melanoma, which is a highly immunogenic tumour. Following that, there has been a range of papers on kidney cancers, prostate cancer, brain tumours, bowel cancers and on and on. These approaches have been mostly used in Stage 3 and 4 cancers and have gone through Phase 2 clinical trials and some have gone through Phase 3 clinical trials. To obtain results in these kinds of patients is indeed encouraging. For example, in prostate cancer

there has been a study with hormone resistant prostate cancer with bony secondaries, with between 30–40 per cent of the trial population showing a significant result. This doesn't always mean complete remission, but certainly means increased median survival time.

In our own experience, as we see mostly Stage 4 cancers, complete remission in a majority of our patients is unusual, but increase in median survival time is often seen and we have a number of Stage 4 cancers now in complete remission following a cytotoxic tumour killing programme followed by a dendritic vaccine. This is especially gratifying, as no significant side effects have been noted from the use of dendritic cell therapy vaccines. A theoretical possibility would be the development of an auto-immune disease and in auto-immune disease the cell mediated immune response is overly powerful and directed at a particular tissue in the body, such as in multiple sclerosis it is directed at the cells making up the myelin sheath of peripheral nerves. However, this has not been observed so far as a side effect in the use of dendritic cell vaccines.

The future
Most clinical trials in dendritic vaccines have been done on patients with advanced disease. These patients have some degree of immuno-suppression from the cancer itself and as a result of conventional treatment programmes, particularly chemotherapy. Immunisation strategies using dendritic vaccines are most likely to be beneficial when applied to patients with low levels of tumour present. However, we have seen complete responses in patients with significant tumour load, so it is worth using dendritic vaccines in many Stage 4 patients.

It is likely in the future that eventually all patients with cancer following a tumour killing approach such as surgery, radiotherapy and chemotherapy, may then go on to have a dendritic cell therapy vaccine. This is particularly likely, as prospective studies have been carried out which look at recurrence in cancer and associated this with cell mediated immune function. In round terms there's a 50 per cent increase in tumour recurrence in cancer patients if their cell mediated immune function is low. This situation is commonly seen following chemotherapy, which depresses immune function. We measure this by looking at levels of a particular cytokine, that is a protein messenger which governs one of the parts of the immune system to do with cell mediated immunity, called Interferon Gamma. We measure Interferon Gamma at the gene expression level. This means we measure the messenger RNA as it comes off the chromosome, to then make Interferon Gamma, which then stimulates cell mediated immune function. We have done hundreds of such tests on all the common cancers and generally after chemotherapy we find Interferon Gamma levels at less than 50 copies per microlitre of plasma, the normal range is 5,000–10,000. In many cases the only way of normalising Interferon Gamma, we have found, is to detoxify the patient from their previous chemotherapy using high dose intravenous vitamin C and then the Interferon Gamma will often respond to measures to stimulate its activity, such as the use of medicinal mushrooms, known as proteoglycans preparations and a range of other possible approaches. Therefore I would advise any patient following a conventional treatment programme, to save the urine and deep freeze it during the time of maximal tumour cell destruction and to look into having a dendritic cell therapy vaccine made, as this lessens the chance by approximately 50 per cent, of tumour recurrence. Just stimulating the immune system is too crude, in dendritic vaccines you stimulate the immune system to recognise specific tumour associated antigens; that is the key. General immuno-activation may not work, it has to be specific against *that* particular tumour, in *that* particular patient. If readers are interested in further scientific papers on dendritic cell therapy vaccine, look on the Dove Clinic website (www.doveclinic.com) there are a range of papers and a research section on that website.

31 Antineoplastons – a non-toxic treatment for cancer?

The work of Dr Stanislaw Burzynski

Chris Woollams

In 1970 a young Polish research scientist, Stanislaw Burzynski M.D. PhD arrived at Baylor College of Medicine in Houston, Texas as Assistant Professor.

His prime interest, an interest that he had cultivated since his time as a graduate student, was urinary peptides (short chains of amino acids) and their anti-cancer activities.

He had originally noticed a difference in peptide content between the blood and urine of healthy people and that of cancer patients. The fact that fascinated him was that normal healthy individuals had much higher levels of certain peptides and that these peptides not only helped in the process of communication between cells (and thus identification of rogue cells by the immune system) but were also known to possess the ability to stop cancer growth *in vitro*. Similar studies at Leeds University had shown the presence of these, but no follow up analytical work was done with them.

Quite early on in his work he concluded that these peptides somehow helped the immune system in its work, whilst also affecting the unique biochemistry of the cancer cell. He managed to isolate about 120 peptide fractions, amino acid derivatives and organic acids for his studies. These he termed antineoplastons, and he prepared two mixed 'active packages' – formulae – both produced synthetically. Both 'mixes' were active against cancer tumours.

It is now clearly understood that, in cancer, as the ras gene can be read and cause a cancer signal to be made (genes that cause cancer are called oncogenes). It is also known that another gene (*p53*) normally suppresses tumours (and turns off the cancer process) but somehow fails in a cancer patient.

Burzynski showed that antineoplastons both turn off the ras gene **and** restimulate the *p53* suppressor, and he thinks of antineoplastons as 'switches' turning some things off and others back on. They provide the messages to tell the genes to act. Without enough of these crucial peptides a cancer is made more likely.

Antineoplaston peptides are made in various parts of the body but primarily in the liver and the kidneys. Two types exist, ones with a very specific activity for specific tissues, and others that have broad scale activity for a wide variety of tissues. Hence his two original 'action' packages.

A cancer patient has a double problem. They make far less of certain peptides than are needed (probably because the genes that control them are poisoned by modern toxins or diet); and also the cancer cell sends out messages to tell the kidneys to excrete them, thus protecting itself.

In case you don't know, peptides are short chains of amino acids, whilst proteins are long chains of more than 30.

The FDA acts
And then it all went pear-shaped. Burzynski's discoveries were at first applauded and he was offered a more junior post but in Baylor's Department of Pharmacology – a job he turned down. Almost immediately his research grant was withdrawn and he was left outside of 'the system'.

In 1983 he applied to the FDA for new drug permits for antineoplastons but was turned down. A lengthy legal battle then took place which included the FDA raiding his offices.

Since there was no statute in Texas preventing him from 'treating' patients with this essentially non-toxic solution, he set up shop for himself. However the US District Court then banned him from shipping his product across state borders. Since he couldn't stop patients taking product back to their homes in other states, he was subjected to Grand Jury investigation and eventually tried on over 70 charges. One by one he beat all of these and 14 years later the FDA and the District Court gave in. An important part of the defence was that these antineoplastons worked!

Brain tumours
In 1991 a group of investigators from the National Cancer Institute went to the Burzynski Research Institute in Houston and reviewed his 'best 7 cases', where patients with astrocytomas —spelling and glioblastomas had mainly experienced complete responses to the 'drugs'. The NCI recommended a Phase II clinical trial, which began in 1993 and was overseen by such eminent people as the Mayo Clinic and Sloan-Kettering Cancer Centre. Only 9 people were followed and the report concluded that the results were insufficient to recommend antineoplastons for a wider use.

Burzynski was extremely unhappy especially when he discovered that the doses used had been far lower than he was using with his own patients. Indeed he had a letter published stating that the levels used were previously established by him to be ineffective!

Meanwhile he undertook his own studies. In one study of 36 patients (all with brain tumours and some of multiforme levels) he produced evidence for the following:

9 (25%) had a complete response i.e. disappearance on an MRI scan.

7 (19.5%) had a partial response i.e. more than 50 per cent reduction on MRI scan.

12 (33.3%) were stabilized.

In his report Burzynski noted "the general consensus in the medical community is that such tumours cannot be cured by chemotherapy, and the response rate is only modest". However Burzynski achieved a response of over 50 per cent, i.e. 16 of his 36 patients.

Dr Burzynski continues with his efforts and currently has over 70 patients in full clinical trials now overseen by a more agreeable FDA. He has also recently won FDA approval for an amino acid 'mix' for home use, but he stresses that this is by no means in replacement for his therapy.

The future
Currently researchers in Kurume University, Japan and Imperial College, London are also exploring the effects of antineoplastons, not just with all types of tumours, but with diseases such as Aids too.

Certain genes have been identified and linked to a number of cancers; others are specific to a certain type of cancer. Burzynski and the Japanese are studying which genes are blocked, and which are over active, with which cancers. It is early days but the full picture may be less than 10 years away and it could have wonderful results. The MD Anderson Cancer Center in Houston, which confirmed Burzynski's initial antineoplaston theories, is world-renowned and they are clear that all the exciting developments in cancer cure lie outside of chemotherapy nowadays.

Recently, Burzynski has developed 12 'active' formulae and believes that far more active packages will be developed in the future. Indeed he believes antineoplastons will eventually become a mainstream treatment for all cancers.

At the end of the day, notwithstanding Professor Pilkington's work on Clomipramine, there is currently no effective brain tumour chemotherapy drug, largely because the blood-brain barrier is primarily there to prevent just such a chemical entering the brain. Nor is there adequate research on non-toxic natural therapies, but clearly these will be far more likely to address problems within the brain. Thus it is likely that the only successful treatment for brain tumours will be 'natural!

But looking beyond to other cancers, the potential is enormous, because cancer patients are clearly deficient in certain peptides. The only problem is that if their production cannot be restimulated (and this probably means finding a cause for the lowered production in the first place) the peptide mixes have to be taken by the patient indefinitely.

Dr Burzynski could be just another brick in a wall of failure. Somehow we doubt it. In which case he could be on his way to a Nobel Prize with his pioneering, non-toxic treatments.

We wish him well in his efforts.

32 Hands on healing

Madeleine Kingsley

icon April 2003

Craniosacral treatment: hands-on help to healing
Alternative therapies sometimes seem mysterious and even slightly alarming to those of us not in the know. Craniosacral treatment is no exception. 'Something to do with the brain and the lower spine?' you might hazard. 'Something slightly bone-crunching, since it's practised by specialist osteopaths?' On the contrary, craniosacral treatment is a gentle, hands-on technique designed to re-balance the stressed body and encourage its own innate powers of healing. Craniosacral osteopaths believe that the flow of spinal fluid in and around the nervous system creates its own body rhythm, distinct from, but no less vital to, health than your heartbeat or breath. Through their hands, cranial osteopaths can 'hear' this rhythm and its subtle changes beneath the bones and membranes of the human body. They don't use their hands to manipulate; they palpate the head and body so lightly that even restless babies benefit and begin to sleep sweetly after treatment.

So how can the technique help those with cancer? 'By dealing' says Nicholas Handoll, a practitioner and teacher at the Sutherland Cranial College 'not with disease or syndrome, but with whole body health. Cranial osteopathy allows the body to make changes that will improve its mechanical function and instigate the fine tuning that makes it operate more effectively.' 'We do not diagnose, offer a cure or any substitute for conventional surgery, chemo or radiotherapy' stresses Philip Owen who practises in South Manchester. 'But we can help restore wellbeing to newly diagnosed patients and enable natural healing after hospital physicians have done their work. Physicians in the medical professions concentrate on disease. Osteopathic physicians concentrate on health. I believe that, given the right encouragement, the body is capable of immense regeneration and that there is health down within us all.'

When somebody discovers they have cancer, says Philip 'There's a huge shock to the system that can hit them like a ton of bricks. Usually that shock stays with them for a while and can be felt, to the palpating hand, as a tension within the system. That in itself can be detrimental to the patient's physiology. It's quite rare for members of the medical profession to look on cranial osteopaths as being of help in this traumatised situation, though I think it will come. So most people I see at this stage are either having treatment with me already or come through word of mouth. A woman with breast cancer, for example, who has already been through mammogram, biopsy and confirming consultation is now very worried. At this stage I would choose not to treat the cancer-affected area at all. There is no proof one way or the other, but one is very careful indeed not to run the risk of increasing the spread, by stimulating the circulation around the chest. I can, however treat the general condition of shock. That woman may need support in her tissues; she may need the whole body gently rebalancing to increase her state of wellbeing and address some of the fear and tension. This stage is not going to be an easy ride for anybody with cancer, but bringing those fears and tensions to the surface so that they may be able to talk about them (which in itself can bring relief) is better for health than burying them deep.' Philip Owen takes a detailed history of all new patients, who also receive an appropriate medical or osteopathic examination. Each actual treatment takes about 30 minutes and usually involves palpation of the sacrum, legs, pelvis, abdomen and chest before Philip balances the head.

After hospital treatment
Cranial osteopathy can relieve the effects of tissue damage or scarring particularly after radiotherapy and/or surgery. Says

Philip: 'Very often after a mastectomy or lumpectomy, the tissues in the upper thorax, at the bottom of the neck and the diaphragm appear in a state of trauma and hypertension. They don't seem able to relax or function. By releasing the tensions in those areas we can revitalise those tissues which helps considerably not only in the healing process but in lymphatic drainage and supporting the immune system. Emotionally too, we can help: patients often seem to regard the areas that have been operated or subject to therapy as almost foreign to them, and craniosacral work is a way of reintegrating that part of the body with the rest. I'm working with one woman who recently had a lumpectomy with lymph glands removed too, and treating her for a swollen arm and armpit with tightness around the chest. She feels much better after each treatment.'

Principles of the Founding Fathers

Modern craniosacral treatment developed from the work of pioneer osteopath Dr Andrew Still. The son of a travelling preacher, Still was an American civil war veteran who lost three children to meningitis and one to pneumonia. Seeking kinder medical methods than bleeding, blistering and purging, Still drew on alternative practises of the day such as bone setting, hydropathy and homeopathy to research a new way of healing – manipulation to improve circulation and correct altered mechanics. Soon 400 people a day were travelling the Wabash railroad for treatment at his first School of Osteopathy at Kirksville, Missouri. Still's philosophy of medicine focused on the unity of all body parts, on exercise and good diet, a belief that the musculoskeletal system is a key element of health, and that the body is naturally self-healing. Still died aged 89 in 1917. Still's student William Garner Sutherland developed the idea that the skull was not a rigid bony structure, but composed of parts that move and shift (a little like the earth's tectonic plates) to allow the rhythmic fluctuation of fluid beneath.

This business of balance

Cranial osteopaths talk about a state of 'good physiology' when the whole body is in balance left and right, top and bottom, front and back, inside and out. 'This balanced situation helps the immune system, helps the tensions around the central nervous system, aids wellbeing' says Philip. 'In other words it's like a car going down the road not having to travel with the handbrake on.' If that handbrake is on, then a cranial osteopath will 'hear' it through his hands. 'We use our hands' says Phil, 'to feel very subtle changes in the body's tissues and the body's mechanisms. By gently putting your hand on the surface of the body, and more or often than not this includes the surface of the skull, it is possible to feel that gentle, rhythmical fluid movement. This is thought to arise from the movement of cerebro-spinal fluid around the nervous system. It's quite separate from pulmonary respiration and separate, too from the cardiac pulse. It's a unique pulsation that carries its own feelings and is affected if a blockage arises. In other words the cranial osteopath can make an assessment of the patient's vitality and wellbeing and of stresses in the system by feeling this pulse.' Philip says he would never seek to take control of his patients or the symptoms he perceives. Hands-on palpation is much more subtle than that: 'If anything I see myself as a servant who works with the pulse and the fluids around the central nervous system to allow the body itself to release any blockages. For the practitioner it's a very passive process: I listen with my hands and through them I'm actually accepting all sorts of information. The body itself will direct the treatment, guiding you to areas that need the work.'

Seeing through the hands
How does a craniosacral osteopath recognise the body's trouble spots? 'Think of a soldier out of step in a marching platoon' says Philip. 'Your eye is guided to what doesn't look harmonious. Your hands are the tools that give you a visual picture of what is going underneath them. To return to the motoring metaphor, it's rather like a car mechanic listening to an engine. He can hear whether it's the engine that doesn't sound right or whether it's the tappets, the exhaust or the fan belt – he focuses in on the noise that doesn't sound normal. When holding somebody's head there is a feeling of normality – or not

– and if the answer's not, then I'm asking why not?' After treatment the tuned body operates more efficiently like a tuned motorcar going along the road more sparkily and using less fuel to go the distance. Says Philip 'I worked with a lady who had cancer of the parotid gland – the gland in the corner of the jaw. She had surgical removal, followed by radiotherapy.

This left her with weakness in the side of her face because of a damaged facial nerve, but she also had constant headaches and a feeling of tightness in the operated side of her head. She had an altered sense of smell and taste and felt really quite wretched. Her whole head felt totally out of balance – one half of her brain felt very tense and traumatised, almost like a cricket ball, whilst the other side had more the feel of a football. By allowing the fluids around the central nervous system to rebalance themselves I enabled the cricket ball to regain its football feel. This lady immediately felt so much better in her optimism, in her aches and pains, her ability to sleep and to start getting back to some sort of normality. That's so important. Treatment shouldn't just be about saving lives; it's also about quality of life.

For Philip Owen the beauty of cranial osteopathy is that it makes patient treatment possible at many different levels. 'There's the osseous or bony level, the membranous level and the fluid level. Then there's the bio-energetic level and also a spiritual level that you can tune into with individual patients. Illness sometimes allows people to take notice of that other part of the body that has previously been ignored – the spiritual side. It can point you in the direction of things about yourself beyond the superficial and material. And that's the silver lining in the cloud.'

33 The power of prayer

Ginny Fraser

icon November 2003

'Prayer is not an old woman's idle amusement. Properly understood and applied, it is the most potent instrument of action.'
                                               (Gandhi)

However sceptical or non-religious we may have been in the past, for many people the challenge of cancer is a spur to investigating or re-engaging with the spiritual aspect of our natures. Often the experience of cancer can have a transformational impact – causing us to become more truly ourselves, more connected to our own values and life purpose and more in touch with a sense of the spiritual.

Frequently people who are sick will call upon prayer to help with the challenges they face. But does prayer work, or is it just a panacea for the desperate? Does praying actually have a physiological effect or could it be just the placebo at work?

Dr William Kelley, an American working in the field of nutritional and metabolic therapy, urged his patients to trust in God, to read the bible and to pray. He believed a positive attitude could play an enormous part in helping to kick out disease. And at Duke University Medical Center in Carolina, doctors have noticed that patients with a God live longer than those who neither believe nor pray regularly. Doctors are now conducting research into this discovery.

There are two types of prayer – that which the individual does for themselves, and that which is received – either knowingly or not – from others. Numerous studies show that in the former case, those who pray contemplatively or meditate – in both Western and Eastern traditions – can positively influence their health. There are many possible explanations for this, depending on your beliefs.

First, those with strong religious beliefs of various traditions believe that by asking for healing through prayer, a loving and omniscient deity will respond. For many this is an unquestionable belief – important and hugely valuable to those who hold it, but impenetrable to those who don't.

Secondly, there are points of view that do not require faith to explain the effectiveness of prayer. The act of prayer requires the supplicant to become quiet, release tension and let go of stress. This in itself has a positive physiological effect. Dr James Le Fanu, medical correspondent in the Daily Telegraph describes an extraordinary piece of research by Professor Luciano Bernardi of the University of Padua. "There is a marked similarity in the physiological effects of chanted yoga mantras and the repetitive Latin of the Rosary Prayer, Ave Maria. ... Surprisingly, they have a common thread, with the Rosary's strong repetitive element having been introduced to Europe by the Crusaders who took it from the Arabs, who had in turn borrowed it from the Tibetan monks and yoga masters of India. Professor Bernardi found that the reciting of the Rosary and yoga mantras slows the respiratory rate to six breaths a minute, which coincides with the rhythmic oscillation of nervous impulses controlling the heart rate. This synchronicity of respiratory and heart rates boosts oxygen in the blood, while improving circulation to the brain."

There have also been developments in the last ten years or so that are bringing together the findings of science with what the mystical traditions have been teaching for centuries, which is based on sound physiological principles. These are so compelling that in the US alone there are 80 medical schools which now run courses for exploring the role of religious practice and prayer in health. The relatively new science of Psychoneuroimmunology looks at the relationship between our thoughts and emotions and our bodies. Scientists have demonstrated that when we have a thought or feeling our brain produces neuropeptides, substances that allow brain cells to communicate with each other. Other cells in the body – most significantly the immune system – have receptors for these neuropeptides, and respond accordingly. As Deepak Chopra, a medical doctor and international speaker on the mind/body connection, says, "Your immune system is continually eavesdropping on your internal dialogue." In his audio programme, *Magical Mind, Magical Body*, he describes how different emotional states produce different chemical changes in the body. For example, tranquillity produces the natural equivalent of valium in our systems; nervousness produces adrenalin; and excitement produces interleukins, which, when manufactured chemically are hugely expensive anti-cancer drugs. He suggests a ride on Magic Mountain at Disneyland (so long as you like that kind of thing!) as an enjoyable and cheap way of producing these powerful chemicals – naturally!!

Thirdly, prayer activates hope. Research by Greer on coping styles shows that those who react to a cancer diagnosis with hopelessness and helplessness have a much lower chance of survival than similar patients with a fighting spirit.

Being prayed for
The second aspect is that of receiving prayer. There have now been numerous studies on this subject, perhaps one of the most well known being conducted by cardiologist Randolph Byrd and published in 1988. Byrd's work took place with coronary care unit patients and was scientifically rigorous using a randomised, double-blind protocol. Over ten months, 393 patients in the unit were – with consent – admitted to a prayer group (192 patients) or a control group (201 patients). They were prayed for by Christians outside the hospital. Neither the doctors nor the patients knew who was receiving prayer.

Although when the study began the patients were of around equal state of health, over time the patients receiving prayer showed much better recovery rates than the others. The prayed-for patients were five times less likely than control patients to require antibiotics and three times less likely to develop pulmonary oedema. While twelve of the control patients needed intubation to help with breathing, none of the prayed-for patients did.

Another impressive study was conducted more recently in 1998 by Dr Elisabeth Targ at the California Pacific Medical Center in San Francisco. Her study (again a double-blind experiment) was conducted with patients with advanced AIDS. Those patients receiving prayer had six times fewer hospitalisations, which were also of a significantly shorter duration than those people who received no prayer. Even Dr Targ herself was surprised, "I was sort of shocked," she said in an interview with ABC News, "In a way it's like witnessing a miracle. There is no way to understand this from my experience and from my basic understanding of science."

Yet another study is by Dr Mitchell Krucoff at Duke University Medical Centre in North Carolina. He studied the effects of prayer on patients undergoing cardiac procedures such as catheterisation and angioplasty. His findings show that patients receiving prayer have up to 100 per cent fewer side effect from these procedures than people not prayed for.

A leading researcher and writer in this field is Dr Larry Dossey, who has written extensively about the power of prayer. On his website, he cites examples from the plant and animal world. When bacteria are prayed for they grow faster; when seeds are prayed for, they germinate quicker; when wounded mice are prayed for they heal faster. He says "I like these studies because they can be done with great precision, and they eliminate all effects of suggestion and positive thinking, since we can be sure that the effects are not due to the placebo effect. "

So if it isn't the placebo effect, what the heck is going on?

An explanation that is gaining more and more scientific veracity is the idea that rather than being separate individuals, each one of us is connected energetically – as suggested throughout the aeons by mystics of many traditions. Deepak Chopra is an eloquent speaker on this subject. He describes us individually as waves that are part of an ocean of consciousness, and gives the example of our breath to explain this. Oxygen is the foundation of all our tissues, and as we breathe in and out we are literally building our bodies. He claims that in our bodies there are around a million atoms that were once in the bodies of Christ, of Gandhi, of Leonardo da Vinci. We are exchanging our bodies with the body of the universe all the time. In fact, 98 per cent of the atoms in our bodies are exchanged within a year. We are connected. And our thoughts are powerful. In this way, the prayers of a nun in a convent in Ireland, or a monk in a temple in the Himalayas, or a rabbi at the Western Wall in Jerusalem can energetically influence – for example – a cancer patient in a UK oncology ward. Chopra says "What physicists are saying to us right now is that there is a realm of reality which goes beyond the physical …. when in fact we can influence each other from a distance." It is a view that is also held by Larry Dossey, who proposes on his website that "consciousness is not confined to one's individual body. An individual's mind may affect not just his or her body, but that of another person at a distance, even when that distant individual is unaware of the effort."

So if you are a religious believer, all of this simply gives some scientific background to what you already believe to be true. If you are a sceptic, this latest research shows there are undoubtedly healing forces in nature that science is only beginning to understand. Whichever camp you come into, prayer is effective and is an important element in the healing journey.

34 'John of God'

Catherine Woollams

icon July/August 2004

As many people know my daughter, Catherine, had a grade 4 Glioblastoma. She was first diagnosed three years and two months ago in late April 2001. Off the record the 'experts' gave her 6 months to live. They have since told her there is little more they can do for her. Back in 2001 a young man approached me at Epsom Races. His mother, a healer, had had a patient who had been 'cured' by a healer in the Amazon jungle going under the name of 'John of God'. Shortly afterwards another person in contact with our **icon** *office told us that she had taken her husband there for treatment and it was, quite simply, a life changing experience. So immediately I hit the internet and, after overcoming my initial cynicism that a man from the Amazon jungle could have a highly polished web site, I passed the information on to Catherine and her mother. Three years later in May 2004 Catherine and her mother visited John of God', also known locally as 'The Entity'. Chris Woollams*

Of all the thoughts and help that came up when I was diagnosed with a grade 4 brain tumour, this was probably the most strange. Following Dad's e-mail, Mum read up about 'John of God', a healer based in Brazil and, 2 years later, thought it would help if she sent my picture and details to him. One day, whilst sitting in Caffe Nero in Chelsea, Mum suddenly appeared with a letter claiming that 'the entity' was apparently already helping me and that we should go to him very soon. As you can imagine, we have tried most things to date, so this seemed another harmless yet positive step. The cost for ten days including all meals, hotels and the treatment was only £900 plus flights, so even this did not seem excessive.

We flew first to Rio de Janeiro and had a few days of very enjoyable R&R. Then, we flew to Brasilia, the new capital, which by contrast has no personality at all. But we did meet all of our fellow 'patients'. There were 15 of us, all with very different aliments from cancer to muscular dystrophy. Everyone was really friendly and warm.

Next we boarded our coach and were taken to Abidijana and to our 'possada' – a very basic bed and breakfast. Once we had had lunch and had met our hosts Robert and Catrina and their daughter Natalie, we were taken to La Casa. This is absolutely beautiful; there is a small shop, a tiny café and then the main building where you wait to see John of God, plus a beautiful view-point from which to meditate and three crystal healing beds. La Casa is also decreed to be so holy that we could only wear white clothes; all things black being viewed as bad. Immediately your shoulders unwind and you relax – it's a truly stress-free setting.

That afternoon we waited in the main room before being taken in a line through to see 'John'. This main room was surrounded by people 'in current' – this term essentially signifies lots of people meditating in an area alive with energy. The queue is very long; I had my step-father in front of me and my mother behind. As we reached John he immediately took my hand and in Portuguese told us that I was to be operated on in the morning and that both my helpers had to be 'in current' for me. In the hall there are TV screens showing 'operations', some of which involve being cut – yet bizarrely no blood emerges. I was terrified.

The next morning at 7 am I went for my two crystal healing bed sessions. This was gorgeous; you simply lie on a bed under the crystals with your eyes shut listening to some relaxing music for 40 minutes. Even this feels like you are being healed.

Next came the operation. At 8 am we were walked through the main hall and taken into a third room for prayer. In here, we were asked if we wanted a physical or invisible operation. I chose physical but because I had had radiotherapy, chemotherapy and a recent operation it was felt that I'd be better with an invisible one.

The operation was equally fascinating. You sit and place your right hand either over the specific and damaged part of your body or over your heart if the illness is general. You have your eyes closed and listen to a man talking in Portuguese. For me it was amazing. When I was first on the crystal healing beds, I had seen white light but had thought that I was going a little mad. But then I was 'operated' on and I could actually feel my head moving inside!

Two other patients, David and Sue, were given physical operations. David has bone cancer all over and had only been given two months to live. He had what I can only describe as a triangular metal instrument (which he said he couldn't even feel) stuck up his nose. However when the instrument was removed from his nose he immediately passed out!! Sue, who has muscular dystrophy, was told to relax and she too immediately passed out from all the treatment pressure to which she was subjected.

After all this we were helped outside – I was shattered – we were photographed and taken back to our posada where we were put to bed and served with special soup that they make fresh at La Casa. You have to eat the special food they provide three times per day along with their prescribed herbs which are also given three times a day after the food. Abstinence from pork, alcohol and sex is essential!

For the next 24 hours I slept. It was as if I had had surgery back in the National Hospital for Neurology. I had some very bizarre dreams but apparently this is very normal when you subject yourself up to this energetic environment.

By Friday afternoon I was again placed 'in current', this time for four hours. The weekend was for relaxing and sleeping. By now we were all getting along very well and games of cards had started. The game, hearts, was never ending.

The weather was gorgeous so sun bathing and reading were also the norm. Below the house there is the most beautiful waterfall, where you go to wash away any bad energies and spirits. On Tuesday we were allowed to go to the waterfall specifically to wash away the bad dreams we had all been having. This, in itself, was amazing – we walked down to this beautiful but cold waterfall and were each asked to step into the falling water and wash ourselves. Invigorating, healing, stimulating and cleansing.

On Wednesday it was back to 'the current' in the morning and then seeing John in the afternoon. So we queued up to see John. He was telling everyone that they were fine; but when it came to me apparently I wasn't and needed another operation! I was quite down about this as I was literally the only one who needed another session but then again by now I had this compelling feeling that I was in the best place for it.

So on Thursday morning I was up early and back in for my second 'operation'. This felt even madder as my head was swirling before I even got into the room. For the next 30 minutes I could feel so many things that I was exhausted when I left. I slept for the next 24 hours with some horrible dreams. When I appeared for breakfast on the Friday morning I have to confess that I felt fantastic and totally relaxed. It was shortly afterwards that the black eye started to develop – exactly as it had when I had had surgery in London!!

A week after your operation you must get rid of your 'stitches'. To do this you have to put a glass of water by your bed and pray to God to remove your stitches that night. The next morning you would then drink the water and your stitches would dissolve too.

I have to confess that I am not particularly religious and this visit to Brazil was not an obvious thing for me to do, but it has been both stimulating and amazing. I have never before felt so in touch with my body and its healing processes. At the centre they repeatedly told us that healing was 50 per cent them and 50 per cent you. I am now convinced that this is true.

So here I am back in London feeling great. I am still having other treatments like Photo-dynamic Therapy and Metabolic Typing but who knows. I haven't been officially scanned at St Thomas' Hospital yet but David, who had all over bone cancer, has just had his psi reading done and it is lower than you, or he, could ever imagine!

So although I can't yet give you any scientific readings on my health, I can tell you that I feel amazing and fortunate. Frankly it was such a friendly experience and I know I have made friends for life.

Catherine died on Friday, October 22nd, 2004, a few months later. She was bright, beautiful and brave right to the end.

Appendices

Appendix I
Parallel reading

Everything You Need to Know to Help you Beat Cancer

A complete, easy to read 'bible' on the basics of cancer, from causes to possible 'cures'. With details on surgery, chemotherapy and radiotherapy plus a host of complementary therapies.

Tel: +44 (0)1280 815166 or via the Internet: www.iconmag.co.uk

The Tree of Life: The Anti-Cancer Diet

An easy to read book about what foods you should include in your diet. Foods that protect and help the fight against cancer In simple English but underpinned by research studies, scientific papers and Nobel Prizes.

Tel: +44 (0)1280 815166 or via the Internet: www.iconmag.co.uk

icon magazine (Integrated Cancer and Oncology News)

This magazine covers everything you need to know to help you beat cancer. It is delivered bi-monthly, free to over 100 top hospitals and oncology units in Britain. Donors of over £30 to our charity CANCERactive may receive 6 issues free to their home address in the UK.

Tel: +44 (0)1280 821211

Appendix II

Contacts

Charlotte Gerson
The Gerson Institute
1572 Second Avenue
San Diego
CA92101
USA
Tel: +1 619 685 5353
Website: www.gerson.org

Dr N Gonzalez
36A East 36th Street
Suite 204
New York
NY10016
USA
Tel: +1 212 213 3337
Website: www.dr-gonzalez.com

Dr Contreras
The Oasis of Hope Hospital
P.O. Box 439045
San Ysidro
CA 92143
Website: www.oasisofhope.com

Dr Julian Kenyon
The Dove Clinic
Hockley Mill Stables
Church Lane
Twyford
Nr Winchester
Hants
SO21 1NT
Tel: +44 (0)1962 718000
Website: www.doveclinic.com

Hoxsey Clinic
Bio-Medical Center
615 General Ferreira
Colonia Juarez, Tijuana
B.C. Mexico
Tel: +52 664 684 9011
Website: www.cancure.org/hoxsey_clinic.htm

Gerald Green
53 Downlands Close
Bexhill-on-Sea
East Sussex
TN39 3PP
Tel: +44 (0)1424 218683 (after mid-day)

Dr John Millward
Southbourne Natural Health Clinic
102 Southbourne Road
Bournemouth
BH6 3QQ
Tel: +44 (0)1202 424833

Mr Tom Greenfield
Tel: +44 (0)1227 761000
Website: www.nature-cure.co.uk

David Broom
Hurn Forest Clinic
40 Wayside Road
St. Leonards
Ringwood
Hants
BH24 2SJ
Tel: +44 (0)1202 874149
E-mail: safesup@btconnect.com

Professor Geoff Pilkington
Director of Research, School of Pharmacy & Biomedical Sciences
University of Portsmouth
St Michael's Building
White Swan Road
Portsmouth
PO1 2DT
Tel: +44 (0)2392 842116
E-mail: Geoff.Pilkington@port.ac.uk

Dr David Walker
Bio-Res-Med, SA DE CV
PO Box 111
San Carlos
Sonora 85506
Mexico
Tel: +52 622 226 0390
E-mail: dlwalker@prodigy.net.mx

Rada Pharma
E-mail: www.radapharma.ru

Dr Bill Porter
E-mail: www.clttherapy.com

Dr Stanislaw Burzynski
Burzynski Clinic
9432 Old Katy Road
Suite 200
Houston
Texas77055
Tel: +1 713 335 5697
Website: www.cancermed.com
E-mail: info@burzynskiclinic.com

Elizabeth Brown
Tel: +44 (0)20 7603 2902
Website: www.gentlepowers.com

Bill Wolcott
www.healthexcel.com
Sheri Dixon
Metabolic Typing England
E-mail: metabolictyping@ntlworld.com

Peter D'Adamo
Website: www.dadamo.com

John Boik
E-mail: john.boik@ompress.com

John of God
Website: www.johnofgod.com

Dr Paul Layman
Tel: +44 (0)1202 814755

Appendix II – Contacts

Nutritional Cancer Therapy Trust
Central Office
Skyecroft
Wonham Way
Gomshall
Surrey
GU5 9NZ
Tel: +44 (0)1636 612707
Website: www.defeatingcancer.co.uk

Dr Etienne Callebout
72 Harley Street
London
W1G 7HG
Tel: +44 (0)20 7467 8348
E-mail: medsec@tenharleystreet.co.uk

General information
All other information – call +44 (0)1280 815166 or visit www.iconmag.co.uk

Appendix III
Contributors

Madeleine Kingsley
Madeleine Kingsley (MA Cantab) is a freelance journalist specialising in health, literature, relationships, TV and celebrity features. Three times runner-up magazine features writer of the year, she has contributed to The Daily Telegraph, The Times, SHE, Cosmopolitan, Country Living, Harpers & Queen and Hello! magazine. She is also an experienced couples counsellor with Relate and works on their behalf with teenagers at risk of school exclusion. 'I am particularly committed to working with Chris Woollams' she says 'because he intends to leave the world better than he found it – and that's what I too have hoped in some small way to do.' Madeleine is married with three grown children and lives with thousands of books and a few horses in the Yorkshire Dales.

Ginny Fraser
Ginny Fraser has been dealing with melanoma for eleven years, most severely three years ago when she was diagnosed with tumours in her brain, lung, spleen and stomach. Her extensive research and commitment to taking responsibility for her own health through many approaches (including the Gerson Therapy, B17, surgery, Rife machine, radiotherapy and intensive detoxes, supplementation and more) has led to her wellness today. She works as a writer, coach and facilitator around the world, specialising in coaching with people diagnosed with cancer. Email ginnyf@dircon.co.uk for more information.

Melanie Hart

A prolific writer and celebrity interviewer, Melanie Hart has worked as a journalist and commissioning editor on some of the UK's leading magazines – as well as writing a book about working mothers. Since moving to Brighton, with her husband, Chris, and children, Natalie and Lucas, and hearing Chris Woollams speak, at a Neways' convention in 2002, she has become very interested in health and well-being. A regular contributor to **icon** magazine, she is passionate about spreading the word about cancer prevention "there is so much we can do to help ourselves" to anyone who'll listen.

Elizabeth Brown

Endorsed by Harley Street consultants, Elizabeth Brown has the ability to get to the heart of an individual's health problem. She is able to identify the root cause behind ill health – or simply what might be preventing an individual from functioning at optimal levels. With over 30 years' training in subtle energies, Elizabeth is able to pinpoint the causative and contributory factors – whether they be environmental or electromagnetic; food allergies or chemical toxins; nutritional deficiencies; or more subtle energies residing in the home or individual energy field.

More information can be found on her website
www.gentlepowers.com

Dr Paul Layman

Humour is one of God's gifts, and I thank her for it! Sometimes when I am writing, this little imp surfaces, and the most serious issues dissolve into playfulness. If I didn't laugh at some of the Doctors Dilemmas (catchy title of my new book) I've got into over my 35 years of medical practice, I would have gone more insane than I actually did. Happily, I woke up from the delusions and now know what Shakespeare meant "We are all actors on a stage".

Appendix II – Contributors

Dr Julian Kenyon

Dr Julian Kenyon directs the Dove Clinic for Integrated Medicine. He has a wide interest in the integration of complementary treatments and conventional approaches in cancer. (See www.doveclinic.com).

He is the founder Chairman of the British Medical Acupuncture Society and the founder President of the British Society of Integrated Medicine. He is particularly interested in encouraging a broader debate on the integration of complementary and alternative medicine into conventional medicine.

Dr Geoffrey Pilkington

Graduated with a BSc in Biological Sciences and PhD in Neuropathology and began his career as a lab technician in 1968. Worked and studied at the Royal Free Hospital Medical School, the Institute of Neurology at the National Hospital for Nervous Diseases, London, the Middlesex Hospital Medical School and the Institute of Psychiatry, King's College, London where he was Professor of Experimental Neuro-oncology before joining the University of Portsmouth in the summer of 2003 as Professor of Cellular and Molecular Neuro-oncology and Director of Research in the School of Pharmacy & Biomedical Sciences. He is currently running two clinical trials to evaluate the potential of mitochondrially-active drugs and bioflavonoids on brain tumours in collaboration with King's College Hospital, London.

David Broom

David Broom has practiced as a medical herbalist and allergy tester for over 20 years. He incorporates many aspects of naturopathic medicine into his practice and has worked at some of the pioneering clinics in this field. For seven years he was Executive Director of a charity clinic in Bournemouth and now practices in Hampshire and Dorset. More recently he is working on projects for growing organic herbs and vegetables and recommends the use of raw juices, herbs and sprouted seeds for the treatment and prevention of disease. David lectures to many groups including students at the local university and local doctors. He and his wife, Judy, work together at their naturopathic clinic at Hurn Forest near Ringwood in Hants.

Gerald Green

Came into medicine at age 45 when life-threatening asthma and emphysema left him in a wheelchair. Whilst in hospital he read extensively looking for alternative treatments and ended up taking a combination of herbal remedies. Immunology and herbalism that saved his life then became his life. Later he also suffered coronary disease and high blood pressure – again which he treated naturally. Meanwhile he worked closely to help people with auto-immune diseases like Crohns, ulcerative colitis, lupus, MS, etc. The cancer treatment came when his own brother was diagnosed with primary prostate cancer and multiple secondary tumours, an anti-candida diet was found to be very successful. He credits his German grandfather (a Professor and scientist) with handing him down a genetic brain!

Dr Robert Jones

Dr Robert Jones took a First in Natural Sciences at Cambridge. His entry into cancer research in 1959 signalled the beginning of a life-long commitment to solving the cancer problem. In 1974 he discovered that interference with the energy metabolism of tumour cells underpinned control of the growth of malignant growths and could cause their destruction. His findings have been published in over twenty papers. The Phenergan treatment described here exploits this original concept and represents the latest advice. His persistent attempts to persuade the MRC and Cancer Research UK and its forerunners to hold clinical trials have been consistently ignored.

To order more copies of this book

Tel: 44(0)1280 815166

Fax: 44(0)1280 824655

E-mail: enquiries@iconmag.co.uk

icon magazine
(integrated cancer and oncology news)

For the latest information,
breakthroughs and news on
cancer prevention and cure,
see icon magazine

For a free trial copy ring:
Tel: 44(0)1280 815166

EVERYTHING YOU NEED TO KNOW TO HELP YOU BEAT CANCER

by

Chris Woollams

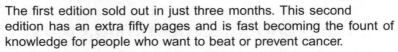

The ultimate guide for people who have cancer and anyone who wants to prevent it.

The first edition sold out in just three months. This second edition has an extra fifty pages and is fast becoming the fount of knowledge for people who want to beat or prevent cancer.

All the causes, all the possible 'cures' from antioxidants to herbs, from liver cleanses to hormones. Plus tips and integrated plans for those facing surgery, radiotherapy or chemotherapy.

This book really is the cancer bible, yet remains a very easy read in straightforward, non-jargon English.

"As you can imagine, I have been sent books, magazines and articles from all over the world, and I want to tell you that your book is head and shoulders above them all. It's informative, practical and really down to earth. It's brilliant."   GEOFFREY BOYCOTT

"Brilliant. There is so much information in the book. I just couldn't put it down."   T.O. (Sheffield)

"This book fulfils an unmet need, it is easy to access and understand, and gives basic information all the way from surgery to nutritional supplements for cancer. This is a truly integrated book and deserves a wide readership."

DR JULIAN KENYON
Medical Director of the Dove Clinic for Integrated Medicine,
Southampton and London

Tel: 44(0)1280 815166
Fax: 44(0)1280 824655
E-mail: enquiries@iconmag.co.uk

THE TREE OF LIFE

2nd edition

The Anti-Cancer Diet

by

Chris Woollams

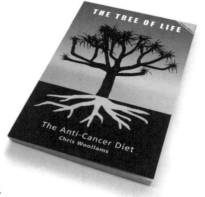

Can one book really change your life?

This new book is revolutionary.

It details all the foods and nourishment you should actually add into your diet to increase your odds of beating cancer.

A simple, easy to read book. It's a book of addition and so quite unlike all those other diet books that tell you what you can't eat.

This book uses real scientific research to explain exactly what foods you dare not leave out of your diet. Miss it at your peril.

With shopping tips, menus and recipes, this book is a must for anyone wishing to know how to eat to beat cancer.

"Chris has done it again. This book looks at the science of beating cancer through diet, and then turns it into something really easy to read and use. He's even produced a shopping trolley of foods to buy and some sample ideas and recipes. Truly wonderful."

DR A.P. (London)

Tel: 44(0)1280 815166

Fax: 44(0)1280 824655

E-mail: enquiries@iconmag.co.uk

OESTROGEN
THE KILLER IN OUR MIDST
by
Chris Woollams

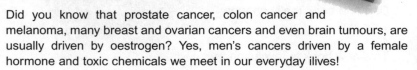

"This book is amazing – it told me things I had no idea about"   Dr J.H. (Salisbury)

Did you know that prostate cancer, colon cancer and melanoma, many breast and ovarian cancers and even brain tumours, are usually driven by oestrogen? Yes, men's cancers driven by a female hormone and toxic chemicals we meet in our everyday ilives!

Some specialists believe 90 per cent of solid cancers are hormonally driven and 90 per cent of these we prove are driven by oestrogen. And this is true for both men and women,

Most usually this is a **breast** cancer but it can be **prostate** cancer, **colon** cancer, **melanoma**, a **brain tumour** or **ovarian** cancer.

Without a doubt the 'driver' is invariably an oestrogen.

Chris says: *"This book is a very important book for anyone with a solid tumour. It is meant to be very easy and quick to read, but to clearly cover the facts and suggest what action you might take to amplify your orthodox treatment. Things most doctors simply do not tell you. It will also save me a lot of time, hormonally driven cancer is so common I have often had the same conversation five times in just a few hours!"*

Oestrogen: The Killer in Our Midst is a self-help book for all those wishing to beat or avoid hormonally responsive cancer.

"It's easy to read and with a checklist of action points. It pulls all the information together in a usable way."   E.T. (Hertfordshire)

"I think it's invaluable for anyone, male or female. It covers everything from cutting oestrogen excesses out of your life to the use of natural progesterone. I didn't realise that there is so much you can do."   P. F. (Limerick, Eire)

Tel: 44(0)1280 815166
Fax: 44(0)1280 824655
E-mail: enquiries@iconmag.co.uk

CANCER
YOUR FIRST 15 STEPS
by
Chris Woollams

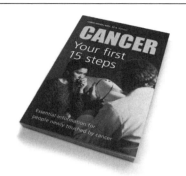

Just been diagnosed with cancer and don't know where to start?

This book provides really essential information for people newly diagnosed with cancer, who want to improve their odds of beating it.

A simple guide to help you prepare an integrated (wholistic) programme of treatment around the orthodox medical skills of your doctor.

We have developed a serious plan – incorporating the **ACTIVE 8 programme** – to enable you to start immediately and take every possible proven step to improve your odds of beating cancer.

A 100 page book that tells it all. A good total cancer programme can increase your odds by as much as 60 per cent.

Tel: 44(0)1280 815166
Fax: 44(0)1280 824655
E-mail: enquiries@iconmag.co.uk

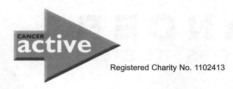

Registered Charity No. 1102413

CANCERactive is a new charity with three important points of difference.

- First, it brings you the WHOLE TRUTH ON CANCER TREATMENTS: all the up-to-date facts about every researched therapy that might be of help to you. From surgery to supplements; from radiotherapy to exercise; from chemotherapy to photodynamic therapy. We don't show bias, we just lay out the facts so you can choose.

- Second, it is dedicated to helping people build an INTEGRATED treatment programme, to maximise their chances of survival. Books, a magazine (**icon**) and an easy-to-follow website are all packed with information and our own research is planned.

- Third, it aims to take the PREVENTION message where it matters, into schools and to parents.

BECOME AN ACTIVIST – JOIN THE FORCE

For just 50 pence per week you can join the FORCE, and receive **icon** posted to your home, a monthly e-newsletter, discounts on health products and a whole lot more.

 "Everything you need to know to help you beat cancer."

Now no one need die of ignorance

Tel: 44(0)1280 821211
Fax: 44(0)1280 824655
E-mail: enquiries@canceractive.com

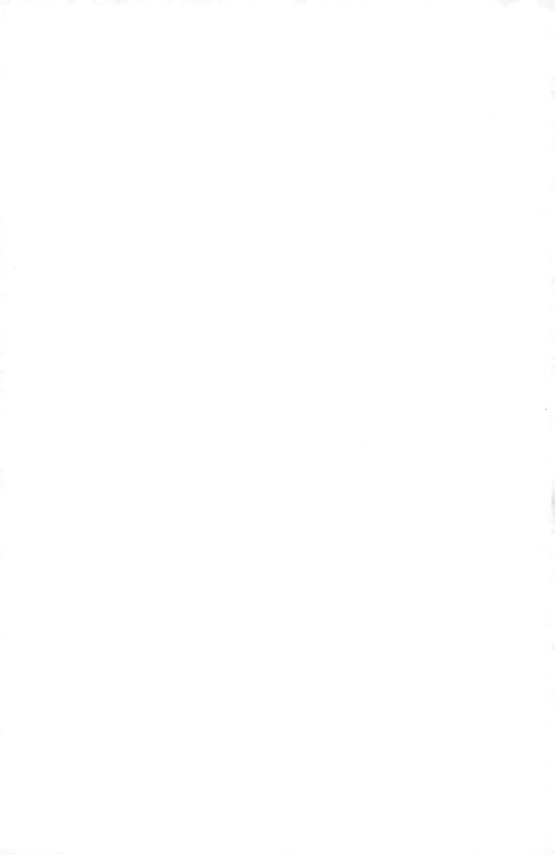